About the Author

Susan Kolb is a medical doctor with a specialty in plastic and reconstructive surgery. She has treated thousands of women with complications from breast implant surgery, and her practice has emerged as an international healing center for women with breast implant disease and other immune disorders. Her medical practice routinely incorporates state of the art surgical technology with holistic medicine and spiritual healing.

She graduated from Johns Hopkins University, received her medical degree from Washington University School of Medicine and completed her post-graduate education in general and plastic surgery at Wilford Hall Medical Center. She served as a surgeon in the United States Air Force, specializing in the treatment of burns, hand reconstruction and cosmetic and reconstructive surgery. Dr. Kolb is a member of the American Society of Plastic and Reconstructive Surgeons, a Fellow of the American College of Surgeons and is certified by the American Board of Plastic Surgery. She is a founding diplomat of the American Board of Holistic Medicine and a member of the American Holistic Medical Association.

Dr. Kolb is the director and founder of Millennium Healthcare, a holistic medical center; Avatar Cancer Center, an alternative cancer treatment institute and Plastikos, a holistic plastic surgery center.

THE NAKED TRUTH ABOUT BREAST IMPLANTS:

Call 1 (770) 457-4677

To order by mail, send check, money order
or credit card number to:

Plastikos

4370 Georgetown Square

Atlanta, GA 30338

United States of America

The
Naked Truth
About
Breast Implants

From Harm to Healing
A Spiritual Healer's Journey as a
Plastic Surgeon

Susan E. Kolb, M.D., F.A.C.S.,
A.B.H.M.

The Naked Truth About Breast Implants

© 2010 Susan E. Kolb

ISBN- 13: 978-1-935079-29-3

Published by
Lone Oak Publishing
SAN 257-4330
5531 Dufferin Drive
Savage, Minnesota, 55378
United States of America

CONTENTS

Foreword

This book is a testament to two important journeys of discovery which merge in the person of Susan E. Kolb, M.D.

The first is the recognition and definition of an important, modern, and environmentally caused new disease, which according to the rules of naming medical disorders is best called siliconosis. Dr. Kolb has made major contributions to this recognition and is one of a limited number of physicians qualified to bring these matters to more general attention. She prefers the equivalent term, silicone implant disease, which conveys to the afflicted patient a more direct statement of cause and effect.

The second journey is even more remarkable: Dr. Susan Kolb experienced the same adverse effects from her own silicone based mammary implants that impacted literally hundreds of thousands of other women.

This book is timely. Against a great deal of research and clinical evidence in the peer reviewed literature in many fields, some dating to before 1950, the American Food and Drug Administration partially reversed its incomplete moratorium on silicone gel content silicone mammary implants in 2006. The ban, imposed by FDA Commissioner David A. Kessler, M.D., J.D. in 1992, was based on such issues as prevalence of rupture with release of silicone gel and oil to elsewhere in the body, fibrous deformation of the chest wall, and a high risk for replacement far short of stated claims of product longevity. What was not taken into proper account was the immunogenicity of silicone. Had it been, so-called saline content devices would have fallen under the moratorium as well. It is the contact of the outer surface of the silicone shell that stimulates the immune and inflammatory response to which are later added the cogent problems of infection, biofilm formation and scar contracture.

Although controversial at the time, and contested strongly by implant surgeons and even more strongly by the manufacturers of these alien devices, the partial ban of silicone implants had a remarkable counter effect. The frequency of implantation of saline content silicone devices rose substantially for the rest of the decade.

After consultation with basic scientists at the University of Tennessee, in particular the then medical director of the Memphis Pathology Laboratory, David L. Smalley, Ph.D., and my then clinical chairman (Obstetrics and Gynecology), Frank W. Ling, M.D., and others, I began a clinic to explore the effects of implanted silicone devices of all kinds, not just mammary prostheses, in February 1996. The timing was in response to the evident lesions formed in the tissues surrounding the devices, the axillary and other lymph nodes and a complex matrix of systemic signs and symptoms new in the health experience of hundreds of women. What was unexpected at the time was the rapidly increasing number of women coming to clinic with adverse effects from their saline content silicone devices.

It was immediately obvious that most of them did not understand that the phrase "saline implants" was a deliberate simplification by the manufacturers, the spinmeisters and some surgeons, to bypass the uncomfortable and inconvenient truth they were basically silicone devices which happened to contain saline rather than other, more liquid silicones. Dr. Kolb describes this accurately and effectively later in this book.

Now that many aspects of the restrictive conditions of the partial moratorium have been removed, we are on the verge of a new epidemic wave of anterior thoracic scarring, chest and axillary deformations, device rupture and migration of small amounts and lighter weight silicones throughout the body, all with their attendant and often vigorous immunological and neurological consequences.

This book, written with clarity from her experience, both as patient and as surgeon and with the wisdom gained from her hundreds of patients, is a cautionary tale for the near and distant future. What comes to the fore are the dysfunctional reviews of science practiced at the FDA these past ten years or so and the innate conservatism of many physicians to reject what is new, no matter how strong the evidence.

Medicine as practiced is a disconnected receptor system for information in which those with vested financial interests have the power to force the conversation away from basic truths, even to attempt to discredit those physicians and researchers with abundant data and no personal axe to grind, to use the common metaphor of a past generation.

Dr. Kolb's record, as both an implanting and an explanting surgeon, shows her to be a clinical researcher of the finest type, and as a woman afflicted by siliconosis, is unassailable by those forces and interests.

Her abilities as a surgeon and a caring physician were the two reasons, during my active clinic years, 1996-2002, I referred more patients to her than to any other explant surgeon. This book, which so well displays the double journey she has undergone, now with a deep understanding of the nature of the disease and how best to help her patients enter the healing process, justifies completely the confidence I had in the late 1990s. She touches on the problems of silicone disease as one of many now emerging environmental threats to human health, some of which, like siliconosis, are due to alien chemicals in the human body.

This book is neither an exposé nor a diatribe. It is a call to allow the self correcting scientific method and process, based on data, not opinion, to be applied to those now emerging disorders of the modern world. The same must be said of the now re-emerging problems of siliconosis. It is the diary of a pilgrim bearing the professional burden of deep knowledge and the agony of her personal experience.

D. Radford Shanklin, M.D., F.R.S.M.
Emeritus Professor of Pathology,
Laboratory Medicine, and Obstetrics and
Gynecology, University of Tennessee, Memphis

Preface

In the physical realm, things are not always as they seem. Life is a school for spiritual mastery, and sickness in the body contains lessons for the health of the soul. Indeed, the soul may receive many gifts through the process of healing: insight, compassion, integrity, discernment, greater self-awareness and enhanced intuition, just to name a few. If we accept the lessons we are given and learn what they are intended to teach us, we inevitably find healing and grace.

This book will serve those who incarnated to learn discernment and those who came into the physical realm to learn to follow their internal guidance, for that is my path as well. Those of us on this path have a choice. We can choose to trust our intuition and follow our internal guidance, or we can choose to give up our connection to what is alive in us and abdicate control over our lives to an external authority.

When illness strikes, it demands that we make that choice. We can choose to listen to outside advisors in the world of medicine instead of the "still, small voice within." If we do this, we may find ourselves on a downward spiral toward progressively deteriorating health and chronic illness. A person who is unable to discern the voice of their inner guidance may follow this path to its ultimate end: suicide or death, often from infectious disease or cancer. Someone on this path may never know the cause of their decline until they experience their life review. At that time they will find out that the responsibility for their health belonged to them.

If they choose to listen to their internal guidance, however, that still, small voice will guide them step-by-step toward the truth of what is slowly eating away at their health. They will not only find out the cause, but will also find effective treatments for their condition. And in this search, they may find themselves choosing a healthier lifestyle. They may also find validation of their intuition. For many, this validation opens a world of spiritual empowerment and healing of old wounds. Many will drop the archetype of victim when they realize they have a choice in how they view the world.

When we see the world and ourselves from a different vantage point, we can project a different future, not only for ourselves, but also for our children and all the generations that follow us. We can break long-standing patterns of the dance between victim and victimizer. We can rise above the worldview of duality into unity consciousness. When we realize that we can become one with that part of consciousness that is projecting our reality onto the screen of time and space, we can begin to consciously co-create our lives by changing what we project.

Acknowledgements

The Naked Truth about Breast Implants is a synopsis of a chapter in the history of medicine. Perhaps the lessons not learned with round one of the silicone saga may be learned during round two. The Food and Drug Administration has returned silicone breast implants to the market after a fifteen-year moratorium. Now a whole new generation of women will have an opportunity to learn discernment and to follow their internal guidance when they find themselves descending into a chronic illness that the medical community refuses to acknowledge.

Therefore, I would like to acknowledge the governmental regulatory agencies and the corporations manufacturing silicone breast implants, without which this book and the spiritual lessons it describes would not be necessary. I would also like to acknowledge that portion of the medical profession that has thus far failed to determine the cause and treatment of the hundreds of thousands of women made ill from their silicone breast implants, and who chose instead to deny the existence of a problem that they have helped to create. If the medical profession had chosen a different path, this book and the spiritual lessons it describes, would not be necessary.

On a lighter note, I would like to thank my editor, Martha Caldwell, for her dedication and talent as an editor and writer. She not only encouraged me to tell my story, but also helped and encouraged my patients to tell their stories and has given voice to the spiritual lessons they learned from their experiences. Martha also encouraged the book to look beyond the breast implant controversy to other areas where technology meets industry. Her grounding in spiritual principles, as well as her ability to see the larger picture, is appreciated and is reflected in the book.

I would also like to thank Jo Ann Sadowski, my friend and transcriptionist, for her dedication and help with the project. I would like to acknowledge the stability given to the medical and surgical practice of Plastikos Plastic and Reconstructive Surgery and Millennium Healthcare, from the combined efforts of my talented and loyal staff members, Karen Vaughn, R.N., Practice Administrator, Pam Fife, R.N. Head nurse of Plastikos Surgery Center, Glenda Holcomb, Accounting, Nadya Dhanani, Front Desk Supervisor and Homeopathic Doctor, as well as Dr. Richard Clofine, Dr. Bradford Gould and Dr. Mike Greenberg of Millennium Healthcare. Without the help of these dedicated medical professionals, I would not be able to handle the volume of patients who have come to us seeking medical and surgical care for the complications of breast implants.

I would also like to acknowledge the extraordinary work in progress of Pamela Jones, M.D., whose story is included in the book, for her creation of the nonprofit Human

Adjuvant Disease Corporation and its website http//www.freewebs.com/implants which has been helping women understand breast implant disease and find help for their problems for four years. I would also like to thank my patients who generously shared their stories in this book as well as the spiritual meaning of their journey through this illness. Finally, I would like to thank my spiritual support group, Stephen Yancey, EMT, and Sheilagh Moister, R.N., for their love, support, and guidance.

Introduction

I am a medical doctor who is uniquely qualified to tell this story because I have a specialty in plastic and reconstructive surgery, as well as extensive training in holistic medicine. Furthermore, both silicone and saline breast implants have been in my body, and I confronted the health challenges such prosthetic devices can produce. While my story is very personal, it also reflects the experience of hundreds of thousands of other women. I have waited patiently for the correct time in my life, as well as the right time in the world, for this information to come forth.

The story I tell involves multinational corporations, public health concerns and governmental organizations that have betrayed the very people they are charged with protecting. Suppressed research, legal battles, government hearings, political corruption and corporate greed are part of this saga. Yet it is also about healing, for it contains the promise that those involved will learn greater responsibility. Sometimes we all have to learn the hard way.

Despite the fact that hundreds of thousands of women with breast implants have fallen ill with "mysterious" symptoms, most doctors have not only failed to diagnose and treat their condition, but they have actively denied that their illness even exists. Despite the efforts of breast implant support groups[1] on the Internet to educate women about the dangers of these devices, large numbers of women remain seriously ill and believe what their doctors routinely tell them: that their implants are not causing their problems. Meanwhile, my clinic treats patients from all over the world, many of whom have been misdiagnosed with lupus, multiple sclerosis and other autoimmune diseases. What they have is chemical toxicity and biotoxicity from breast implants, which often produce devastating systemic effects in the body.

To make matters worse, in November 2006, the FDA returned silicone breast implants to the market, so the entire fiasco is now destined to replay itself. Even more women will descend into chronic illness and struggle to find proper treatment as they search through the maze of misinformation and denial. Almost daily I receive phone

---

[1] See: http://www.humanticsfoundation.com
http://www.explantation
http://www.breastimplantinfo.org
http://www.toxicbreastimplants.org
http://www.freewebs.com/implants
and http://groups.yahoo.com/group/SalineSupport/

calls from women who have already developed the symptoms of the disease. Symptoms from the newer generations of silicone implants may appear after only a few years of exposure, while the older implants typically took eight to ten years.

The Naked Truth about Breast Implants is not just a story of my personal journey. It is also the story of my patients' journeys from a progressive sickness (unknown to most physicians) to a healthier state — physically, emotionally and spiritually. The common thread in their stories involves the importance of being able to follow their internal guidance. They trust it to lead them out of the quagmire of misinformation and poor medical advice they received. It is a testimony to the resilience of the human spirit.

The treatment protocols I have developed from treating hundreds of women with this disease incorporate state of the art medical technology, including surgery, with many disciplines of alternative medicine and spiritual healing. While our current medical model sees causation of disease only at the level of the physical, I realize that by helping my patients address their spiritual, mental and emotional issues, they not only recover more quickly, but are also better able to maintain a state of health.

I have no doubt that there are many levels of existence outside of our third dimensional constructs of space and time. As we derive reliable means to access them, we achieve a broader view of what we are experiencing at this level. Seen from a higher dimensional perspective, problems or illnesses encountered in ordinary life can serve as vehicles for spiritual growth and human evolution. Healing becomes not only about the body, but also about the recovery of the emotions, mind and spirit.

This multidimensional view of the world gives meaning to what we experience in our ordinary lives. If three-dimensional reality is all that we experience, we live in a chaotic and fear-based world, devoid of higher meaning. We may see no purpose worthy of the suffering and pain we endure. However, the information we access about our current situation from the higher levels not only gives meaning to our lives, but gives us hope for a better future when our current lessons are learned.

In part, the purpose of this book is to introduce this aspect of reality to those who are suffering because of the ignorance of medical, corporate and governmental institutions. My hope is that they can understand some of the lessons involved, not only for themselves, but also for those who deny that their medical problems are related to their implants. I hope to give meaning to the trials and suffering of so many women who trusted the word of their doctors and plastic surgeons.

Many thousands of women were told that breast implants were safe and "would last a lifetime" (as was indicated in the Dow Corning product literature). I hope to illuminate the gifts these women have received through their illness in learning to "go within" in order to solve their difficult health challenges.

This problem, however, is larger and involves more than just breast implants. It reflects a larger pattern and is, perhaps, a major sign of our time. Similar situations exist for users of cellular telephones, food additives and nanotechnology, wherever technology meets industry. The problem, simply stated, is that we fail to adequately test the effect of new products on our bodies prior to their release to the public. As the effect of these electromagnetic energies and substances can be cumulative over time, short-term animal or human studies are inadequate to assess the risk. For example, most scientific studies testing the safety of silicone and saline breast implants were done immediately following implantation, while most health effects tend to develop several years later. This would be like studying smokers who have been smoking for five years or less and concluding that there is no risk of lung cancer from cigarettes.

Once these new technologies are widely in use and the adverse effects become evident, the arena changes. The corporations that developed the technologies are on the defensive as class-action lawsuits spring up. This makes it difficult for the involved companies to acknowledge the health problems they are creating. They find themselves in a defensive posture, and consequently their energy, research and funding goes into protecting their corporate interests. If the same companies were to correct these problems and develop new safety features, they could achieve an advantage in the marketplace over their competitors by helping their consumers. These corrections have not been made because the companies are reluctant to admit there is a problem. Consequently, they are in a legal, financial and ethical bind.

Similarly, government agencies (such as the Food and

Drug Administration and the Center for Disease Control) are ill equipped to acknowledge or study the problem. Indeed, in the case of breast implants, thousands of FDA MedWatch forms, filled out by women who knew they were ill from their silicone gel breast implants, had little impact. The FDA even helped fund a peer-reviewed study published in *The Journal of Rheumatology*[2] that showed that rupture of silicone gel implants predisposes patients to fibromyalgia, but later ignored the study and re-approved silicone implant use after a fifteen-year ban. The National Organization of Women then organized congressional support for a bill entitled "The FDA Scientific Fairness for Women Act" (H.R. 2503), which would require closer regulations of breast implants, but the bill died in committee.[3]

Industry influences within government organizations are problematic. For instance, the testing protocols are usually designed by the industry involved in marketing the products, rather than an unbiased third party. This conflict of interest does not result in sound research. When companies conduct research on their own products, the climate for corruption is ripe. Dow Corning, for example, was aware of silicone's toxic effect from as early as 1954, but this in-house research was suppressed and was only

---

[2] Brown, S. Lori, Gene Pennello, Wendie Anne Berg, Mary Scott Soo, and Michael S. Middleton. "Silicone Gel Breast Implant Rupture, Extracapsular Silicone, and Health Status in a Population of Women." *Journal of Rheumatology* 28 (2001): 996-1003.

[3] "H.R. 2503 [110th]: FDA Scientific Fairness for Women Act (GovTrack.us)." *GovTrack.us: Tracking the U.S. Congress* 14 Feb. 2009. http://www.govtrack.us/congress/bill.xpd?bill=h110-2503

discovered thirty years later as a result of lawsuits brought by those injured by their silicone gel implants.[4] Meanwhile, hundreds of thousands of women suffered the impact of silicone poisoning.

Our current corporate structure dictates that some health care providers, as well as manufacturers of health related products, answer to shareholders rather than the patients they are responsible for treating. Where profit, rather than compassion, is the key consideration in health care delivery systems, an unfortunate enigma arises. Health care institutions are bound to be expensive, ineffective and, at times, even harmful to those they are intended to serve.

At the core of the controversy lies a larger disease. It is a systemic social and spiritual disease that affects us all. The framework for the cure involves the ethical advancement of our institutions: government, medicine, public health, law and business. At this point in our history, we are called to evolve into a more unified state of consciousness and acknowledge the extent of our interconnectedness. We must view our problems from a broader context. We must move as a people from an ego-based concept of ourselves as a merely existing in the physical realm and channel the energies of the higher dimensions into our cultural institutions.

If we fail this test, we may very well not survive as a

---

[4] "Frontline: Breast Implants on Trial: Breast Implant Chronology." *PBS.* 1995-2008. 19 Jan. 2009.
http://www.pbs.org/wgbh/pages/frontline/implants/cron.html

species. Chemical toxicity, left unchecked, could conceivably reach levels that interfere with reproduction or cause significant problems with cancer, immune disorders or epidemics of strange, new diseases. Silicone, chemical and biotoxicity are indicators in an early warning system, signaling a possible future that may lie in wait for our species. We must heed the signs. The importance of intuitive guidance applies not only to our relationship with implants, but also to any substance that we put into or on our bodies. It is only through the concept of our bodies as channels for change that we can revolutionize our institutions and bring healing to our world.

-1-
The Wounded Healer

"Well behaved women rarely make history."
Laurel Thatcher Ulrich

In alchemical lore, the "wounded healer" is an archetype or universal symbol. In keeping with the archetype, the healer is initiated into the sacred curative arts through an ordeal of personal hardship. The ordeal can involve contracting an illness or suffering an injury or an emotional wound. The challenge to the initiate is to journey deep within the psyche to find the means to heal oneself. Thus the edict: physician, heal thyself.

Often the initiate must confront an unconventional illness for which there is no known cure. A person who experiences this type of initiation emerges not only healed, but also transformed, and with an exceptional knowledge of healing. A new path of service unfolds divinely before her, because once the healer finds the remedy for her own ills, she can then use her medicine to heal others.

In retrospect, it was inevitable that I would experience the archetype of the wounded healer. I would have to experience what my patients were going through in order to understand their illness. I would have to confront an illness so unconventional that many doctors would not even believe it existed. I would have to find a treatment by trusting my own internal guidance.

The Early Years

Even as a child, I had a strong sense of guidance. I seemed to know things that other people didn't. Sometimes I sensed things that would happen before they occurred. With strong instincts about people, I was sensitive to emotional as well as physical energies. I was close to nature from a young age and had an affinity with the natural sciences. Gravitating toward medicine, I read books about genetics and biology in grade school. Hours were spent observing life through the lens of my microscope. I tracked animals in the forest and made plaster casts of their footprints. I created three-dimensional animals out of paper that opened up to show their internal organs.

When I was eleven, I contracted pneumonia. While in the hospital, my chest was x-rayed every day, and I believe the chest x-rays during this crucial developmental phase may have interfered with my breast development. Though I can't be certain of the cause, my breasts did not develop normally.

Growing into adolescence, I was not excessively concerned with the size of my breasts. I had other ways to identify. School was easy and I managed to do well with very little effort. In high school I developed strong friendships and belonged to a group of very bright and internationally diverse kids. I had the opportunity to learn about a variety of cultures from close, personal relationships with friends who had lived in many places throughout the world.

After graduating from high school, I attended Johns Hopkins University and majored in premedical studies. I worked summers and nights to help finance my college education. I wanted to get my undergraduate degree as quickly and as inexpensively as manageable, and was on the fast track. My scores on advanced placement exams in high school earned credits in English and calculus, so I already had sixteen college credits when starting Johns Hopkins. Then I took heavy class loads each semester while managing to maintain a consistent A average. Some days classes were from seven o'clock in the morning until eleven o'clock at night without a break. I also worked as a research assistant in my off hours. In spite of my intensely busy schedule, I was thriving.

My spiritual education during my college years was as accelerated as my academic education. By the time I arrived on campus in 1972, I had become an agnostic. During high school I had been so active in church activities that my mother complained about the time I spent there. I was deeply involved in the youth ministry, raising money to fund projects to help underprivileged children. Yet despite having excellent and progressive teachers in the church, my developing faith did not follow the "party line" of mainstream Christianity. I questioned everything taught.

Indeed, the spirit of the times supported a more expansive viewpoint. This was the era of the Civil Rights Movement and the Viet Nam War. The streets of the nation were full of protestors questioning the status quo, and prominent theologians were declaring, "God is Dead" on the covers of national magazines. The youth culture was leading the country in a paradigm shift away from the belief system of the mainstream Protestant Church of my childhood. Society as a whole was heading into a broader, more universal concept of reality. I had also been exposed to many cultures and religions through my diverse, ethnic array of friends, and I found it impossible to believe that any single culture's religious beliefs were superior to another's.

While I rejected some of the ideas of mainstream Christianity, I still had not formed an alternate concept. God as an organizing, creative force was not an idea I developed until later. It wasn't until I began a serious study of biology and saw life under the microscope that I began to consider the nature of God. Through the lens of the microscope, I saw wondrous things. The patterns inherent in the structure of life were undeniable. I saw a magnificent plan behind life and realized that it simply could not happen by chance. No physics would support the theory that life happened as a random incident. There had to be a creative force at work in the design of nature.

An event that happened in my freshman dorm room, however, took me to the next stage of spiritual development. Alone in my room, studying for a test one afternoon, I fell asleep while reading. I woke up from my nap early that evening. The first sensation I was aware of as I opened my eyes was a golden glow filling the room. The entire room was bathed in a soft light that was unlike anything I'd ever seen before, and it obviously wasn't coming from the window. There was an otherworldly quality to it, as if it were emanating from another dimension. I turned around to look behind me, seeking the source of the light, and there, standing beside the door, was a radiant seven-foot angel. The angel was male, with broad wings and a golden sword. I froze in fear for I knew this was no dream.

This "vision" shifted my entire paradigm of reality. Everything I believed was called into question. From that moment on, I could no longer call myself an agnostic and entered into a new level of faith. That experience left me with a sense of knowing that was beyond question.

Years later I had the opportunity to interview Doreen Virtue, PhD, on my radio show. Doreen has written many books on angels[1], and she told me that I have two male warrior class angels as my guardians. Because my spiritual work is to protect the underdog, I need extra protection in my job.

While I was at Johns Hopkins, it never occurred to me to pursue the study of plastic surgery, even though I worked at the Baltimore Shock Trauma unit on weekends. There, the plastic surgeons taught me to sew the tedious multiple facial

---

[1] Virtue, Doreen, *The Miracle of Archangel Michael*. Carlsbad, CA: Hay House, 2008. (For other books by Doreen Virtue, see www.angeltherapy.com).

lacerations that occurred when patients went through the windshield unrestrained, and I received compliments on my handiwork.

During the last year at Johns Hopkins, I worked as a research assistant and was involved in some exciting research in endocrinology. My professors encouraged me to return to Hopkins after medical school and continue to work with them in research there. I was fascinated by the research and had every intention of following the advice of my mentors.

I graduated from Johns Hopkins in 1975 after three years, and my advisors recommended that I go to Washington University for medical school because it had an excellent department in internal medicine. To pay my way through medical school, I joined the United States Air Force Reserves and agreed to serve four years as a military doctor. Of course, I was twenty years old and could not possibly foresee how this decision would affect the course of my life. At the time, I only knew that I needed a way to go to medical school, and I felt guided to pursue that course. Content to trust in my internal guidance, it had never let me down.

I was accepted into medical school at Washington University and found that they did, indeed, have a fine program for the study of internal medicine. They also had one of the best programs in the country for plastic surgery. Many of the founding fathers of plastic surgery had taught there, and several future program directors and important contributors to the field of plastic surgery were on the staff while I was attending medical school.

Intuition

One night around midnight, I was sitting at a table in the hospital cafeteria eating a chili-dog with my friend Barry. We were having a conversation about our future plans, and I suddenly got an intuitive "hit" that I would become a plastic surgeon.

I looked across the table at Barry and said, "I'm going to be a plastic surgeon."

"But you don't know anything about plastic surgery," Barry replied.

"That may be true," I said, "but, nevertheless, I'm going to become a plastic surgeon."

I couldn't explain to Barry how I knew, of course, but from that time forward I was certain I would become a plastic surgeon.

As fate would have it, I was soon offered an opportunity to do research in the plastic surgery department. I spent many hours a day putting together chicken tendons and repairing rat vessels using microsurgery, and spent months participating in research involving microsurgery, wound healing, and the complications of breast implants. During that time, one of the attending plastic surgeons asked me to review the world literature to date on the complications of breast implants and write a review paper on the topic.

This project gave me a firm background, not only in plastic surgery research in the area, but also in contributions from pathology, basic science research and materials research. Such information would be invaluable later when my plastic surgery practice became the Mecca for women with complications from breast implants.

I graduated near the top of my class from medical school at the age of twenty-four and was accepted at the University of Virginia for surgical residency. However, several weeks before I was scheduled to begin work at the University of Virginia, I received orders from the Air Force to go to Wilford Hall Medical Center, a thousand-bed Air Force hospital at Lackland Air Force Base in San Antonio, Texas.

At Wilford Hall Medical Center I embarked on a three-year course of general surgery and then was accepted into a plastic surgery residency. On my first day there, the head of plastic surgery looked across the operating table at me and said, "I don't think women should be doctors." Fortunately, I thrive on conflict, and as a female doctor in the United States Air Force, this particular aspect of my personality served me well.

I served in the Air Force for nine years and emerged with a sense of admiration for people who choose this path. The military is, in many ways, like a small family, and I met many courageous and dedicated people. One of them was my mentor in medical school who had been a prisoner of war for seven years. When he was in the POW camp, he saw so much suffering that he promised himself if he were ever released and allowed to return home, he would go to medical school and become a doctor.

While in the Air Force, I received what I think is the highest compliment a woman in the military can receive from an admiral and former Navy fighter pilot on whom I had just performed a six-hour cosmetic surgery. He had been rescued from a prisoner of war camp and had lost so much weight and experienced so much stress that the skin on his face was extremely wrinkled and sagging. Our hope was that by performing surgery to remove the visible signs of his prolonged ordeal, he would not be reminded of his suffering every time he looked in the mirror. We hoped that after cosmetic surgery he could better put those years behind him and move on. In my mind, it was the least we could do considering the personal sacrifice he had made for his country. As we were leaving the operating room, he began to come out of the anesthesia and regain consciousness. He looked up at my chief first assistant (a female oral surgeon) and me and groggily said, "You girls sure do have balls."

Guidance on the Path

Women get breast implants for any number of reasons, but I have never heard of a woman who got breast implants for the reason I did. Even as a plastic surgeon with very little breast development, I was not particularly interested in breast augmentation for myself. I have never been especially concerned about what other people think of me, so I wasn't particularly susceptible to the societal pressures some women feel to have large breasts. I was also involved in a relationship with a man who had no concern whatsoever about the size of my breasts. As a very busy Air Force plastic surgeon on active duty, I didn't have much time to think about my appearance.

While on leave from the Air Force and on vacation with my family in Venice Beach, California, I made a decision to get breast implants. I wasn't feeling well that day and thought I might be coming down with a cold, so I stayed in the condo after my family left for the beach. I wanted to meditate, thinking that if I could relax and center myself, I would feel better. As I sat quietly, a strong intuitive sense emerged from within, an urge to get breast implants. This was the same intuitive sense that had urged me to become a plastic surgeon, to join the Air Force, and would later guide me to Atlanta, Georgia to establish my practice. I instinctively knew that this was my internal guidance system at work and that this direction would be part of my path. At the time, however, I could not possibly foresee how.

The year was 1985, well before the outbreak of concern that occurred in the early 1990s involving the safety of silicone gel breast implants. I could not even begin to imagine how a journey through sickness and health would be the guiding force in my evolution as a doctor. I only knew that my sense of guidance had always been true.

When I returned home, I called my friend and mentor, who was the chief of plastic surgery at Scott Air Force Base. He promptly arranged for my surgery.

On the evening before surgery, I lay sleeping in my hospital bed when I was abruptly awakened by my mentor's voice. "Get up, Susan," he said, "We have a surgery to do."

I quickly put on my scrubs and followed him to the emergency room where a patient who had suffered a serious ear laceration after an altercation with a tree branch while jogging lay waiting. My friend stood behind me and we chatted while I sutured the ear. After returning the ear to a more natural state, we discharged the patient from the emergency room, and I returned to my hospital bed.

The next morning I went into surgery as a patient, and

my plastic surgeon placed Dow Corning low bleed silicone gel implants under my chest wall muscles. I spent the next few days recovering from the surgery while watching MTV on the hospital cable channel. I then flew back to Wright Patterson Air Force Base, unaware of what lay ahead.

Within a few weeks, I developed a minor but frequently seen complication of breast implants called capsular contracture. This occurs in between five and thirty-five percent of patients receiving breast implants and is caused by hardening of the scar capsule that forms around the silicone or saline breast implant. The implant itself is a Silastic silicone shell that contains either silicone gel or saline (salt water) within the shell. The body recognizes the implant as a foreign body within the first few weeks and puts a scar capsule around the implant.

If this scar capsule remains thin and pliable, the breast implant feels more natural. However, if this scar capsule thickens and contracts because of the scar tissue shortening, the breast implant feels firm and often migrates upward on the chest wall. Not being the ideal patient, I had embarked on a rigorous spring-cleaning of my house during my recovery period and most likely overused my right arm, causing a capsular contracture on the right side. Other than having to avoid certain clothing that would show the asymmetry, this complication caused little problem.

After recovering, I returned to my busy multi-faceted plastic surgery practice with the Air Force. My days were spent performing scar revisions, breast reductions, cosmetic surgeries, burn surgeries, hand surgeries, breast reconstructions, and body contouring surgeries. I established a craniofacial board that helped manage children with facial deformities. I helped plan the surgical hospitals that would be later used in Desert Storm, especially those pertaining to burn care. I was still using silicone gel implants for my cosmetic augmentation or breast enlargement patients, as well as my reconstructive breast cancer patients. I was pleased to have low bleed gel implants available and felt they were a positive advancement over the thinner walled silicone gel implants of the late 1970s and early 1980s. The earlier models were too flimsy and likely to break. They also had the problem of excessive silicone gel leakage through the Silastic shell even before they were put into the patient.

Four years of service to the United States Air Force were over in 1988, and I was guided to Atlanta, Georgia. I joined a thriving plastic surgery practice, but after two years, left to embark on the spiritual quest that opened the door to my study of holistic medicine. During that time I became vegetarian, meditated five to seven hours a day, and worked several times a week with a group of spiritually minded individuals to further develop my intuitive skills, spiritual sight and hearing, healing ability and the gift of quieting the mind to better receive instructions and guidance. This training turned out to be of great benefit when I returned to a surgical practice six months later.

Eventually, I established Plastikos Surgery Center, a medical center with four operating rooms. Plastikos Surgery Center was developed as a holistic center to help restore health to the body, mind and spirit through cosmetic and reconstructive surgery, including hand surgery and laser surgery. As the center began to evolve, three distinct groups of patients began to emerge in my practice. One group consisted of severely injured patients with either facial or extremity injuries from accidents.

The next group had conditions that affected their hands and upper extremities such as tenosynovitis, reflex sympathetic dystrophy and other nerve disorders. These patients were often in severe pain and had very little use of their arms. They had been ousted by the traditional medical system involving Workman's Compensation and were given little hope of recovering. Some of them had been accused of malingering or were told they had nothing wrong with them by doctors who aligned themselves with the insurance companies. They were sometimes spiritually and emotionally broken.

In the third group were patients who were sick from silicone and saline breast implants. These patients, also disenfranchised by the medical community, came from all over the world seeking help for their ills. Typically, their doctors failed to recognize their conditions, misdiagnosed them and often told them that their illness existed only in their heads.

After experiencing positive results with their treatment through Plastikos, my patients began to ask us to provide other medical services, which would include the same holistic and spiritual approaches we used in the surgery center. I founded Millennium Healthcare in 1998 to deliver a similar combination of western allopathic medicine and holistic medicine. Through Millennium, we made available a number of techniques to improve the functioning of the energy body, including Traditional Chinese Medicine, craniosacral therapy, massage therapy, NAET (allergy elimination), chiropractic and osteopathic manipulative therapy, psychotherapy and hypnotherapy. Several physicians who are experts in traditional, as well as holistic medicine are currently associated with Millennium Healthcare.

Our latest addition is Avatar Cancer Center, founded to treat life threatening illnesses such as cancer, AIDS and other viral diseases such as hepatitis. Because these illnesses are life threatening, the treatment programs focus not just on the physical level, but addresses spiritual, emotional, mental and physical issues simultaneously.

Throughout my life, my love of medicine has never faltered. I have continued to read and study both the literature in traditional allopathic medicine as well as spiritual and holistic medicine. When asked to co-host a radio show (and later a television show) on holistic medicine, it was a wonderful opportunity to interview authors and healers on the cutting edge of developments in the field of holistic medicine.

From clinical experience, extensive reading and research, interviews with a wide array of respected experts, and reliance on my own intuition, I began to synthesize a medicine that was not yet in existence for diseases that were not yet recognized. It was through my own initiation as a wounded healer that I truly began to understand the nature of the disease I would need to treat.

Descent into Chronic Illness

As the years progressed, I experienced the gradual onset of an insidious illness. I began to notice increasing fatigue, a more frequent incidence of sinus infections, periodontal disease, alternating constipation and diarrhea, excessive thirst, dizziness, muscle aches, blurred vision, rashes, frequent viral infections, frequent urinary tract infections, left-sided chest wall discomfort, and numbness of my left arm. It was easy to diagnose my medical condition as my waiting room was full of women with the same problems.

Most of the women I was seeing in my practice had implants that were over eight years old. Like me, they had developed the onset of silicone implant disease, often with as many as twenty different symptoms, some of which were nonspecific. Many of my patients had received extensive work-ups costing tens of thousands of dollars with no abnormal findings other than the occasional abnormal antinuclear antibody test (ANA), which was usually discounted.

Some arrived with the usual misdiagnosis of multiple sclerosis or the autoimmune disease of the week or vague, unsubstantiated diagnoses of chronic fatigue syndrome or fibromyalgia. Many were simply considered hypochondriacs by both their physicians and their families. I knew I was not a hypochondriac, and because the silicone gel was leaking out of my left breast implant to a greater degree than the right, many of my symptoms were more prominent on my left side, including my chest wall and arm.

My own implant removal surgery had to be delayed because of an explantation deadline imposed by the 3M

23

legal settlement, which required that women have their implants removed by December of 1996 to substantiate rupture. That month seemed endless as I operated long hours, removing ruptured and leaking silicone breast implants so patients would be able to submit proof of rupture before this deadline.

In January of 1997, I underwent removal of my leaking silicone gel Dow Corning low bleed implants. I asked two of my plastic surgery colleagues to perform the surgery. It had been my practice to remove the scar capsule surrounding the breast implant in a manner that would minimize any leakage of silicone gel outside the capsule. I also felt it was important to remove the entire scar capsule because it was known that retained scar capsules could be a source of complications after surgery as they contained the silicone and the chemicals that leaked out of the defective implants.

When looking at my pathology report after surgery, I noted that very little of my scar capsule had been removed. When I questioned my colleague regarding this, he replied that removing it was too difficult because the scar tissue had adhered to my ribcage. With the majority of the capsule containing silicone gel and associated chemicals still in my chest wall, I knew I probably would have a stormy postoperative course.

I struggled with a progressive illness for the next six months, which threatened my ability to remain a surgeon. However, my determination to keep my practice led me to find detoxification protocols and protocols for the immune system which would work for both me and my patients. Like the archetypal wounded healer, I focused on healing myself.

24

Before my surgery to remove the silicone gel implants, however, I had gone into meditation to ask if I should replace them with saline implants or not. The answer I had received was to replace them with saline implants because "it is not over yet." My initiation as the wounded healer was to continue. The meaning of this very interesting but cryptic internal message was revealed over time. Within the next decade I began to see increasingly more women with problems associated with their saline implants.

Journey to Healing

In retrospect, I realize how important it has been to experience the same things my patients have gone through. I have learned to be more compassionate, to identify exactly what is happening in their bodies, and how to best treat the illness. I was able to integrate allopathic and holistic medicine training with everything gleaned from many leading doctors in the field (through interviews on my radio show).

The resultant treatment protocol has been effective for both my patients and me. When speaking publicly about these diseases, I can first share my own experience and then about the successful treatment of my patients. Not only have I been a physician, but also the patient, which is an additional protective factor as well.

During this period, an Atlanta attorney who represented women injured by their breast implants had extensively researched the science behind the silicone controversy. He provided me with a list of 254 peer-reviewed articles on silicone toxicity. They included chemical, epidemiological, immunological, neurological, pathological, rheumatological and toxicological reports. It was so ironic that the various groups designated by the government to study this problem could ignore such an extensive amount of peer-reviewed literature.

Had I been just a plastic surgeon eager to protect my breast augmentation practice, rather than a breast implant recipient who suffered from silicone toxicity myself, I too might have been inclined to ignore this large body of evidence. As a patient and a surgeon, I knew how much silicone gel had been in my implants when they were placed in my body in 1985, and how much silicone gel by weight remained in the intact breast implants removed in 1997.

Between forty to fifty grams of silicone was missing and was most likely still in my body. Therefore, I researched and read the extensive literature available about the adverse effects of silicone and the chemicals in these implants. This discovery revealed how such chemicals produce toxic reactions that stress the immune, endocrine, metabolic and neurological systems. I also learned treatments that would enable the body to eliminate such toxins.

By the mid 1990s, the Internet was emerging as a powerful avenue for reaching people all around the world and rapidly becoming a source from which patients could gather information on newly emerging syndromes and diseases with which their family physicians were not necessarily familiar. When I wrote an article about silicone immune disease based on my research, it was circulated throughout the Internet and around the world. The article was entitled "Doctor, Are You Listening?"[2]

"Doctor, Are You Listening?" outlined the progression of symptoms many women experience from faulty breast implants, as well as the frustration they feel when they meet with doctor after doctor who cannot diagnose or, worse yet, denies their condition. It also contained part of my own story, including my frustration with implant companies, doctors and health agencies who were somehow incapable of responding to women suffering from this devastating condition. I included my analysis of effective holistic treatment protocols and women from all over the world read the article and recognized their symptoms. Many realized for the first time what was happening in their bodies. As a result of this article, my practice became an international center for women with silicone-related disease.

The Stories of My Patients

Millions of women, as well as their loved ones and families, have been affected by the breast implant controversy. I have witnessed these women's suffering and seen the obstacles they have had to overcome in their efforts to find help and healing. Eight of my patients have elected to tell their own stories. They have generously written the stories of their

---

[2] Kolb, Susan E. "Doctor, Are You Listening?" 1996. *Millennium Healthcare.* 19 Jan. 2009.
http://plastikos.com/documents/DoctorAreYouListeningTheSiliconeCatastrophe.pdf

descent into illness, their journey toward wholeness and the lessons they have learned along the way. Their hope, like mine, is that their stories will enlighten and encourage women who find themselves in similar circumstances.

These women describe their arduous journeys from a progressive sickness unknown to most physicians to a healthier state, not just physically but emotionally and spiritually. These are the stories of women who were challenged to reach deep within themselves to find solutions to potentially devastating health problems. These heroic women have had to overcome enormous odds in their struggle to get to the truth and get well. They describe spiritual guidance and synchronicity that reaches far beyond the realm of the physical. Guidance came to them in the form of dreams, answers to prayers and a sense of inner knowing that they were required to trust. Some of them had to travel great distances from their homes to find the help they needed.

Only those who were able to follow their inner guidance were able to overcome the misinformation by medical authorities stating that silicone and saline implants were not affecting their health. Each of these women, brilliant and beautiful, tells her story of searching for answers. Their stories are both tragic and inspiring. There are, no doubt, still large numbers of women who are seriously ill from their breast implants. But due to the nature of their illness and the effectiveness of the breast implant industry's public relations programs, they are not receiving effective treatment.

My patients arrive from all over the world, often with

misdiagnosis of lupus, multiple sclerosis and other autoimmune diseases. What they have is chemical toxicity and bio-toxicity, originating in and around their breast implants. I suspect we will be seeing even more bizarre diseases in the future, as the chemicals within these implants mix with other chemicals in our food supply and environment to create an entirely new class of disease.

There is, however, a broader context in which to view any problem that we encounter, and the issues surrounding breast implants are no exception. Access to solutions, I believe, can be obtained from a source higher than our third dimensional existence. Indeed, as Albert Einstein said, "No problem can be solved from the same level of consciousness that created it." These women share testimonics of their healing.

Pamela's Story

Pamela's story is remarkable in many ways. First, it shows us the kinds of problems that even a physician educated in traditional medicine can experience in her search to find the cause of an implant related disease. Second, it demonstrates some of the common manifestations of saline immune deficit, especially in the healing period following explantation surgery. Finally, it demonstrates the heroic response so many women facing this debilitating illness find within themselves.

When Pamela first called me in 2003, I had not yet discovered the cause of many of my patients' saline breast implant disease. The diagnosis of silicone immune dysfunction, atypical neurological disease and systemic candidiasis were all correct, but the cause of Pamela's condition was most likely due to biotoxins from her saline breast implants rather than chemical toxicity as we see in silicone gel patients. It would be a few more years before I would distinguish these two diseases.

Pamela tells us in her story that she developed a serious infection after a Florida physician removed her implants. This complication following her surgery required a debridement procedure, which resulted in additional scarring. Through studying the immune deficits I routinely see with this disease in my practice, I have learned the importance of treating these immune deficits in the perioperative period. Fortunately, our patients have been able to avoid the type of serious complications that some plastic surgeons commonly encounter.

Pamela went on to establish the Human Adjuvant Disease Corporation, a nonprofit corporation dedicated to helping patients who are ill from breast implant disease, as well as educating physicians regarding this condition. I am pleased to be involved with her, as she has created one of the most comprehensive websites detailing this information.

Pamela has helped countless women receive the correct diagnosis and treatment. She works tirelessly to connect women suffering from breast implant related diseases to physicians who can help them and support networks who understand what they are experiencing. Pamela, also a wounded healer, has transformed her pain into service for others. (The Human Adjuvant Disease Corporation website is http://www.freewebs.com/implants)

"I had my first breast augmentation surgery in Nassau Bay, Texas the summer before I entered medical school. It seemed as though a lot of women in Texas were going under the knife to have larger breasts. I was a size 34B and had a mild tubular breast deformity which means the lower half of my breast hadn't developed normally. I wanted larger and rounder breasts.

"My boyfriend at the time was a vice president in a major corporation, and he didn't care for my nose or breasts. He told me he would support my decision to have either a nose or boob job. I chose breast implants, but in hindsight, I wish I had chosen a donut breast lift and rhinoplasty instead.

"As a teenager I was told that I was attractive, but I think most of the kids at school noticed that I was smart rather than pretty. I was in Latin Club and played clarinet in the band. I had many friends and always had a boyfriend. Other kids would copy my homework, but I wanted to be noticed more for how I looked.

"I had wanted to become a doctor since I was a child. In college at Ohio University, I majored in biology (premedical program) and won a series of academic honors while I was there. I was active in volunteer work at a family services health clinic and a mental health clinic. I also became involved with The AIDS Task Force and wrote a paper on the state of AIDS and public health. I received my B.S. in 1995, graduating summa cum laude.

"After graduating I moved to Texas to attend chiropractic school, but later realized it was not the right path for me. When I got the opportunity to attend medical school in Belize, I knew that was right for me.

"Like most girls, I was exposed to society's concept of what feminine beauty is at an early age. Barbie™ and Bratz™ dolls do not reflect the average looking female. As girls progress into adolescence, they are exposed to media images of slender females with flawless skin, white, straight teeth, large breasts and full lips. These images may be stored subconsciously in an unspoken and undefined way, which later can lead to a trip to the plastic surgeon's office.

"There is also pressure from men who look at *Playboy* or other magazines and think they would be happier if their girlfriend looked more like the nude model than the way she is naturally. I personally would like to see an issue of *Playboy* printed that lists the surgical procedures and costs next to the naked woman, so men can see how much work each of them has had done to their faces and bodies. I think most of them have been 'enhanced.'

"I remember walking into the plastic surgeon's office for my consultation. There was a large picture of a beauty pageant winner (a former patient) on the wall. I thought that I must have chosen the right surgeon when I saw her stunning photograph.

"During this visit to the doctor's office, he discussed options regarding the type of implants I would have, the placement of the implants, incision sites, and the size of the implants. I showed him photos of Pamela Anderson and told him that was what I wanted to look like. I made an appointment to have the surgery at the local hospital.

"The day of the surgery, I only remember being taken to my boyfriend's convertible corvette in a wheelchair after the procedure. My breasts were bandaged and I was feeling some discomfort. My chest had been inflated with 525 cc saline-filled implants, which were overfilled to 630 cc on the right and 640 cc on the left. The implants were placed in the subglandular position through two very small periareolar incisions.

"Within a few days, the pain subsided and I was astonished when I saw my new breasts. They looked great and were very comfortable. I thought at first they might be too large, but I definitely liked them better than what I had before. I went shopping for new tops and bras to fit my new chest. My new bras were a size was a 34DD.

"Three months later, I left for Belize. I enjoyed

medical school in Central America, except for the school uniforms: a white collared shirt with a khaki/tan skirt or khaki/tan trousers and a laminated name badge with my picture and semester on it. I brought clothes from the States, which conformed to the dress code while at the same time expressing my sense of style. I never wore anything to school that revealed cleavage.

"Even though I was a good student and voted class representative, a female instructor at the university complained to the administration about my shirts supposedly violating the dress code. She said that my button up shirts were too tight on my breasts. In my opinion, I dressed better than most of the other students and my shirts were definitely not tight. I did not want any trouble, so I started wearing loose white collared jersey shirts that I felt looked sloppy.

"I also had a male friend tell me that some of the students were making comments about my chest. I laughed it off and said they should worry more about passing classes than my breasts. Deep down it bothered me, but I always tried to be positive.

"I spent two years in Central America learning about medicine in classrooms and clinics. I moved to England in 2000 where I studied psychiatry at Princess Royal Hospital in Haywards Heath and then moved to Enfield Town where I studied medicine at Chase Farm Hospital until 2001. I really enjoyed it but found it challenging in rotations with some students from The Royal Free and University College Medical School.

"During ward rounds they were always more prepared. I remember asking one of them if he memorized his textbooks before the rotation even began. At least I had the chance to wear suits and dresses in the U.K. instead of uniforms. I enjoyed expressing my style and liked shopping for clothes in Europe.

"In 2001, I moved to Chicago, Illinois to study medicine. A few months later, I noticed that my implants were sagging, rippling and palpable through my skin. I made an appointment to see a plastic surgeon in Chicago. He recommended a mastopexy (breast lift) and exchange of the breast implants. He also discussed additional procedures with me during the consultation and suggested that I bring in photos to show him what I wanted to look like.

"On August 17, I went into the hospital for surgery, including an open rhinoplasty and chin implant under conscious sedation. On September 14, less than a month from the previous surgery and my parents' anniversary, I was in the operating room again for the following procedures performed under monitored anesthesia care: implant exchange (375 cc implants filled to a volume of 460 cc in the submuscular position), an inverted T mastopexy (breast lift), upper lid blepharoplasty and malar (cheek) implants. My surgeon told me that he overfilled the implants to prevent rippling.

"I spent the next few weeks in bed with constant pain. I had a bottle of Vicodin™ on a stand next to my bed and plastic bags filled with frozen peas draped over my face. Within a few months of those surgeries, I was back in the surgeon's office for a dermabrasion procedure to remove scars around my mouth and chin. I talked to the plastic surgeon about my concern over the appearance of my chest. My breasts did not look normal anymore, the nipples were not symmetric, and I was left with raised, red scars. He assured me that the results were very good and that my chest would look much better in another year.

"The following year I graduated from medical school and took a job in Miami, Florida working in research. I had a job, a boyfriend and a social life. It was at this time, approximately ten months after the aforementioned surgeries, when I became very ill.

"One day I was sitting at work, and when I stood up, I felt terrible pain in my knees and elbows that could only be compared to the feeling one may experience if beaten severely with a baseball bat. My speech became labored and slurred. I was very scared and felt like crying with every step that I took.

"I left work that evening thinking that I just needed a little sleep and everything would be O.K. in the morning. But I didn't even make it home. My knees and elbows hurt so badly that I couldn't drive. I went to the emergency room closest to my house. I didn't want anyone at the hospital where I worked to know I was sick.

"Over the next few months, I was in and out of doctors' offices without any answers regarding my medical condition. I developed memory loss, swollen glands, fungal infections in my mouth and nails, and rashes on my inner thigh, groin, neck, and on my left breast. I slept about sixteen hours per day and was too fatigued most of the time to feel like getting out of bed. The joint pain and arthritis persisted. I took prescribed medication, which helped somewhat.

"The memory loss was the one symptom that I was unaware of at first. Others became frustrated when they would tell me something and I couldn't remember, or when they asked me to perform a task and I forgot. I would make espresso and forget to use the carafe so I had to clean the coffee off of the countertop and the floor. I went to the gas station, prepaid, and then forgot to put the petrol in my car.

"I was no longer working and decided at that time to take a course in research. A few months later the wife of the principal investigator of the study I had been working on called and wanted me to come back to work. I couldn't. I couldn't even finish my course.

"In October 2002, I flew back to Chicago for a scar revision procedure on my chest. The surgery only slightly improved the appearance of the scars. I voiced my concern to the surgeon about my implants and told him that I felt pain where the implants were located and that I had other symptoms. He assured me these symptoms were not related to my implants.

"My health continued to worsen over the next year. I went to several physicians in Florida and none of them were able to diagnose my medical condition. Due to the rashes on my groin and swollen glands in that region, I had two pap smears and was told by the doctor that I might have gonorrhea or chlamydia! I was taking pills for problems I didn't even have until the test results came back negative. Besides, my boyfriend and I used condoms, so where would I get an STD?

"Other doctors had different theories about my mystery medical problems. One doctor diagnosed a large red nodule on the back of my neck, larger than the size of a quarter, as psoriasis and gave me a sulfur compound to treat it. He also gave me a pamphlet on exercise and how it was useful for people with depression because I slept a lot. Before the arthritis, I exercised about two hours per day, so I was perplexed at his treatment since I could no longer exercise without experiencing excruciating pain.

"Another doctor explained that as long as I did not have silicone gel implants, I couldn't be ill from the surgeries and he gave me narcotics. Yet another doctor tested me for hepatitis, which I had been vaccinated against and to which I had never been exposed. Eventually I gave up on each and every one of them and decided to do some research on the Internet about my symptoms.

"I read an article previously published in *Glamour Magazine*[1] about a woman with a terrible infection that began with her breast implants. Her symptoms seemed similar to mine. What if it was my implants making me so ill? What would I do? Only a handful of people even knew that I had five implants in my body. The woman in the article had gone to a plastic surgeon named Susan Kolb in Atlanta, Georgia. I decided to reach out to a total stranger and contacted Dr. Kolb.

"Dr. Kolb diagnosed my illnesses as silicone immune dysfunction, atypical neurological disease, and systemic candidiasis. Atypical Neurological Disease and silicone immune dysfunction are components of Human Adjuvant Disease. Dr. Kolb told me that the chin implant, malar (cheek) implants, and breast implants were probably the cause of these ailments.

"In June 2003, a plastic surgeon in Tamarac, Florida removed all of the five implants. I had rippling of the

---

[1] Cool, Lisa Collier. "Could Breast Implants Make You Sick?" *Glamour* Nov. 2000: 247-96.

implants, asymmetry of the breasts, thick raised scarring and asymmetry of the nipples. The left breast implant had completely flipped with the valve on the surface side, which was palpable through the skin. The older incisions were reopened and I had another inverted T mastopexy. During the healing process,

"I developed an infection that became so severe that I had to return to the plastic surgeon's office for a debridement procedure. This procedure involves removing dead, damaged or infected tissue to improve the healing potential of the remaining healthy tissue.

"I remember the first time that I saw myself in the mirror after the explantation. My face looked bruised and puffy and my breasts were bruised and stitched from one end to the other, I collapsed to the floor screaming and crying.

"If someone had told me in 1998 that in five years I would have had four surgeries on my breasts, including two mastopexies, a chin implant and malar implants inserted and removed, I simply would not have believed it. I was told that the breast implants would last at least ten years and that the facial implants would last for the rest of my life. No one told me that my implants could ever possibly make me ill. If someone had warned me, I wouldn't have gone through with any of the surgeries.

"I called the manufacturers of my implants thinking that maybe they were unaware that facial implants or saline-filled implants could make women sick. Quickly I learned that they were not unaware but rather ignoring the problem entirely and ignoring the consumers who had implants in their bodies. The lady I spoke to on the phone at the breast implant company listened to me and told me she had arthritis too but never had implants, so there was no reason for me to think that my breast implants could cause arthritis.

"She didn't take any of the information I gave her down or send me any forms to fill out. She didn't talk to me about how to report my problem to them or the FDA. I didn't even know about MedWatch at the time. I was also told that no scientific evidence existed to prove that implants cause illnesses. I phoned the chin implant manufacturer and told them about my situation. I was told that they could only speak with the doctor who implanted me, not the one who diagnosed or removed my implants or me.

"At this point I felt an obligation to do something to help other women and men with implants or silicone injections who suffered from mystery illnesses and weren't getting any better. I was obligated not only because I was an M.D., but also because I was an injured consumer with information that could be useful to others. About a month after my explant surgery, I founded a non-profit organization called the Human Adjuvant Disease Corporation. We have the best Vice-Chairman. Her name is Susan Kolb and she volunteers tirelessly to help others.

"The Human Adjuvant Disease Corp.. has been helping silicone implant recipients for five years now. Every time I open my e-mail, I read a letter from another victim of the implant industry. Many of them are struggling with a variety of debilitating symptoms, such as joint and muscle pain, fungal, bacterial and viral infections, fatigue, inability to concentrate, memory loss, hair loss, dry eyes and mouth, sores that won't heal, ringing in the ears, alternating diarrhea or constipation, lumps in their breasts or other areas, sleep disturbances and dermatitis to name just a few.

"The list goes on and on. I know many of them are frustrated, depressed, scared, and looking for a compassionate person to listen. They often have children depending on them and are frightened by what is happening to them. They know they are sick, but are being told by doctors that they are suffering from depression. They are often desperate and feel betrayed by doctors who don't listen and implant manufacturers that don't care.

"The most important thing that women realize when they read the site is that they are not alone. They can join a support group to help them with the emotional, mental and physical issues prevalent among women who have this disease. There are doctors listed on the site who do explantation surgery. We list lab tests and costs. There is published research for women to see the types of illnesses that investigators have linked to implants.

"I tell women they can print anything from the site and take it to their physician if their doctors are unaware that such research exists. Unfortunately, sometimes a patient may have to travel a great distance because there is no one in her area to diagnose or treat implant-related illnesses. Sometimes when a woman specifies that she can't travel, I search the yellow pages and call surgeons in her area to assist her in finding the help she needs.

"Compassion is one trait that I have developed from this experience. In medical school I remember seeing a lot of patients with arthritis. I knew the definition of arthritis, the tests to order for diagnosis, and what meds were usually prescribed, but it wasn't until I felt arthritis that I truly understood what it meant. Similarly, because I have suffered so much from implant-related illness, I can well understand and empathize with the women I encounter through my website.

"I have grown spiritually as well. I think that we all have a special gift, talent, or knowledge of something that makes us unique and able to contribute something important in today's society. My gift has been to provide timely, accurate information and support to women who are suffering without remedy. I have the medical and psychiatric training to address the issues they are confronting on a number of levels.

"But ultimately, the breast implant controversy is not an individual problem. Its true resolution rests in the collective society. I think that ultimately the 'social conscience' that Carl Jung described in his writings will prevail over corporate America. According to Jung, the founder of analytic psychology, we inherit a predisposition for certain ideas.

"Humans have a predisposition and potentiality for ethics, which is rooted in the collective unconscious. Specifically, the negative emotion aroused in injured consumers may be lifted up from the collective, leading to justifiable anger and action for social change. Being informed is the basis of our decision-making. Corporations do not have the right to withhold or distort facts and statistics to generate larger profits. They have no right to deny patients the right to informed consent.

Pamela Jones, M.D.
Human Adjuvant Disease Corporation.
http://www.freewebs.com/implants

-2-
A PRIMER ON BREAST IMPLANTS

"The world is a dangorous place, not because of those who do evil, but because of those who look on and do nothing."

Albert Einstein

Breasts symbolize many things to many people: womanhood, motherhood, sexual prowess, eroticism, desirability and beauty, to name just a few. In American culture, breasts are more than just mammary glands designed to nurse infants; they are an integral component of feminine identity. I sometimes joke that in American culture breasts come in two sizes: too large and too small, but mostly too small. Women seek breast enlargement for any number of reasons: from the desire to fill out a swimsuit to pleasing a boyfriend to reconstructing tissue removed in a mastectomy. Invariably, women get breast implants because

43

they want to feel better about themselves.

The History of Breast Augmentation

Clinical breast augmentation procedures were first introduced in the late 1890s when doctors injected liquid paraffin directly into women's breasts. As with any introduction of a foreign substance into the human body, this approach led to unwelcome complications, including infection, hardening of the tissue surrounding the injections and lumps in the breasts. When this method proved unsuccessful, it was followed by attempts to implant glass or ivory balls or other materials. All these methods resulted in problems due to infections and the human body's insistence on rejecting foreign materials.

In the 1920s, surgeons began to experiment with fat transplants. Fat was removed from the buttocks or abdomen and transplanted to the breasts. This procedure was also largely unsuccessful because the body quickly reabsorbed the fat and often left the patient with lumpy or asymmetrical breasts. It also left scars in the areas of the body from which the fat had been removed.

In the 1940s, Japanese prostitutes, believing that American servicemen preferred women with large chests, had their breasts injected with non-medical grade silicone. This practice also became popular in the United States among topless dancers in Las Vegas and other parts of the country where having large breasts could be a professional asset. Silicone injections were banned in Japan in the late 1940s due to serious complications, including infection, chronic inflammation, migration of the silicone to the organs, tumor-like lumps and an association with cancers. In the United States, however, it remained legal until the 1970s.[1]

The 1950s brought the advent of polyvinyl sponge implants. These implants quickly shrank and hardened once inside the body and their complications included infection, inflammation and a link to cancer. Removal of these devices was also problematic and caused permanent disfigurement in some women.

In the early 1960s, Dr. Frank Gerowe and Dr. Thomas Cronin, two plastic surgeons from Texas, developed the first silicone breast implants. Gerowe, who came up with the idea while kneading a plastic bag filled with blood, contacted Dow Corning Corporation and suggested they develop a prototype from silicone. Dow Corning agreed and developed a "mammary prosthesis device" consisting of a Silastic shell filled with silicone gel. The envelope containing the gel was to be surgically implanted underneath breast tissue to enlarge or reconstruct breasts. In 1962, Timmie Jean Lindsey, a 30-year-old mother of six, who initially consulted Gerowe to have a tattoo removed, became the first woman to be implanted. Two years later, Dow Corning took the implants to market.

Silicone breast implant surgery resulted in immediate complications in some cases, such as localized infection, inflammation or capsular contracture. Capsular contracture

---

[1] Leviton, Richard. "Poisoned Breasts." *Alternative Medicine* (November 1998): 48-54.

can occur whenever a foreign substance is introduced into the body. The body reacts by trying to wall off foreign material from the rest of the body by encapsulating it. This means the tissue around the breast implants forms scar tissue, which can sometimes constrict the implants, causing pain and in some cases rupture.

In the two years between the first implant in 1962 and the time the product came to market in 1964, there were no studies or research that could begin to address the effects of silicone leakage on the immune system, a condition that occurs usually over a period of years. Gerowe correctly predicted that in the coming years, thousands of women would want the breast implants he had invented, but what he did not predict was that thousands of lawsuits would be filed against their manufacturers.

In the early years, chemists at Dow Corning saw silicone as a scientific boon. A synthetic compound derived from quartz and sand, it was stronger than plastic and more flexible than glass. It remained stable at both very high and very low temperatures, and it didn't appear to react with many other compounds. In 1947, *Fortune Magazine* predicted that silicone was destined to become a world-class industrial plastic and synthetic.[2]

Over the ensuing years, Dow Corning marketed silicone in products designed to seal buildings, waterproof leather and clean eyeglasses. Their laboratories even created Silly Putty™ out of silicone. Because almost everyone at the time

---

[2] Byrne, John A. *Informed Consent*. New York: McGraw-Hill, 1995: 30.

believed silicone was a biologically inert substance, Dow Corning also used silicone to manufacture medical devices, such as shunts to drain fluid from inside the skulls of children with hydrocephalus, chin and cheek implants, testicular and penile implants, joint replacements and of course, breast implants. Internal company documents, however, later revealed that Dow Corning knew as early as the 1950s that the silicone used in breast implants was "bioreactive, immunogenic, toxic and inflammatory in the human body."[3]

The early breast implant devices often had Dacron fixation patches so that the implant would adhere to the chest wall muscles. These early implants were placed between the chest wall muscles and the breast tissue through an incision on the lower part of the breast called a submammary incision.

In the early 1970s, changes were made in the manufacturing process to create a thinner Silastic shell that encased a more fluid silicone gel, making the implants look and feel softer and more like natural breasts than earlier models. A double lumen implant was also developed that had a saline filled compartment around a silicone gel implant. This allowed the surgeon to fill the outer lumen with varying amounts of saline to better correct mild breast asymmetries or differences in size.

---

[3] Alexander, Richard. "Update On Breast Implants: The New Evidence Against DOW Chemical." *The Consumer Law Page*. 1994. 02 Feb. 2009. http://consumerlawpage.com/article/dow.shtml p. 2.

Plastic surgeons continued to have challenges with capsular contractures, which occurred in over thirty percent of breast implant patients.[4] To help reduce this rate, placement of the breast implant underneath the chest wall muscles was suggested. We found out later that capsular contracture is often caused by subclinical or low-grade capsular infection, so this new position for the implant reduced the incidence of this complication. Placing implants under the chest wall muscles where they were surrounded by vascular muscle rather than less vascular breast tissue was more successful. Breast tissue contains mammary ducts that naturally have low-grade bacterial content, which possibly contributed to infections causing capsular contracture.

Surgeons also began experimenting with different incisions, including one called inferior periareolar, which was placed on the lower aspect of the nipple areolar complex. Although this approach helped to hide the scar, the sensation, as well as the function of the nipple, could be compromised due to inadvertent damage during surgery to the nerves supplying this area. For surgeons who preferred to place the implants either completely or partially under the chest wall muscles, the submammary incision, which is placed just above the natural crease underneath the breast, proved more useful.

---

[4] Unites States. Institute of Medicine. *Safety of Silicone Breast Implants*. Ed. Stuart Bondurant, Virginia Ernster, and Roger Herdman. Washington, DC: National Academy P, 1999.

48

By using this approach, breast ducts, which could contain harmful bacteria, were avoided, and adjustments of the insertions of the pectoralis muscle could easily be made. Later, surgeons would experiment with axillary incisions made in the armpit in order to introduce the implant underneath the pectoralis muscle from above. The main problem with this approach was that adjustments to the position of the implants were difficult to make at the level of the breast fold, and sometimes the position of the breast implant was too high on the chest, giving an unnatural appearance.

Given what we have learned about the role of bacterial and fungal infections around breast implants, it may be best to avoid incisions in areas such as the axilla and the umbilicus or belly button, as these two areas may contain higher levels of bacterial and fungal growth than the skin of the lower breast. Indeed, based on studies, both the FDA and the implant companies have suggested that the approach through the belly button not be performed due to the high complication rate.[5]

In the years when breast implants were first introduced,

---

[5] "FDA Breast Implant Consumer Handbook - 2004 - Breast Implant Surgery & Related Issues." *U S Food and Drug Administration.* 8 June 2004. United States Food and Drug Administration. 31 Jan. 2009 http://www.fda.gov/downloads/MedicalDevices/ProductsandMedicalProc edures/ImplantsandProsthetics/BreastImplants/ucm064263.pdf See also implant manufacturers' websites: http://allergan.ca/assets/pdf/M712-04_Saline_DFU.pdf http://www.mentorcorp.com/pdf/pids/saline_spectrum_ppi.pdf

the FDA regulated pharmaceutical products, but not medical devices. It wasn't until 1976, when Congress enacted the Medical Device Amendments that the FDA began to regulate new devices being brought to market. Since silicone breast implants had been on the market for almost fifteen years, they were "grandfathered" in.

The Silicone Controversy

Meanwhile, many women with breast implants were experiencing symptoms of silicone related health problems, and some were beginning to come forward. In 1977, a Houston attorney for a Cleveland woman won a $170,000 settlement in a lawsuit against Dow Corning, claiming her ruptured implants and subsequent operations caused her unnecessary pain and suffering. This first settlement on behalf of an injured plaintiff received little attention, but it set a precedent for cases that would follow.[6]

In 1984, the case of Stern versus Dow Corning set another important precedent. Maria Stern, a double mastectomy patient, had experienced a range of health related problems including weight loss, hair loss, fatigue and loss of sight and hearing. During the process of discovery for her case, her attorney, Dan Bolton, found several boxes of damning internal company documents in a Dow Corning storage area. These records indicated that Dow's own

---

[6] "Frontline: Breast Implants on Trial: Breast Implant Chronology." *PBS.* 1995-2008. 19 Jan. 2009.
http://www.pbs.org/wgbh/pages/frontline/implants/cron.html

research team had established silicone's toxic effects in laboratory animals, beginning in 1954. Bolton also found a series of internal memos proving that the company was aware of a multitude of complaints from doctors whose patients were suffering the ill effects of silicone poisoning.

In addition, Bolton brought in medical experts who testified as to the possible effects of silicone toxicity on the human immune system. The jury awarded Stern $211,000 in compensatory damages and $1.5 million in punitive damages. After unsuccessful attempts to have the verdict overturned, Dow Corning agreed to pay the settlement in exchange for a "protective order." The final court order kept the embarrassing and incriminating internal documents from becoming public. It also kept them from being examined by the FDA for almost seven years [7]

Throughout the controversy, Dow Corning and other silicone implant manufacturers continued to assert that the implants were safe and carried only minimal health risks for women, mostly involving chest wall problems. Even as they began to settle lawsuit after lawsuit, they never admitted that silicone had a systemic effect on the body or that it could be scientifically linked to the autoimmune and neurological diseases from which these women were suffering. Dow Corning's own research suggested the exact opposite of what company representatives were saying in public. In the 1970s, the corporation reported that silicone

---

[7] Byrne, John A. *Informed Consent*: 96-105.

implants caused no health issues in four laboratory dogs. Years later court proceedings revealed that one of the dogs had died and the other three suffered chronic inflammation.[8]

Court findings also showed that the company received a bevy of complaints from plastic surgeons, who reported that their Dow Corning breast implants appeared oily and seemed to be leaking, even before they were inserted into women's bodies. A company executive sent a memo to the sales staff instructing them to wash and towel dry the implants before showing them to surgeons to conceal the leaking. Dr. Don Bennett left the company during this time, complaining that economic interests were given precedence over responsible medical research.[9]

Thomas Talcott, a senior Dow Corning materials engineer, quit in a dispute over the safety of silicone implants. Talcott later told a newspaper reporter, "The manufacturers and surgeons have been performing experimental surgery on humans."[10] According to an internal company report, Dow Corning research scientists concluded that a preponderance of evidence suggested that silicone produces immune-mediated diseases.[11] Nonetheless, Dow Corning continued to state that breast

---

[8] "What Dow Knew." *Silicone Holocaust*. 02 Feb. 2009.
http://siliconeholocaust.org/whatdowknew.html
[9] Ibid.
[10] Smart, Tim. "Breast Implants: What Did the Industry Know and When?" *Business Week* 10 June 1991: 94.
[11] "What Dow Knew."

implants were safe and did not cause systemic problems in the body.

In June 1988, the FDA changed the classification of breast implants to class III medical devices. This meant that manufacturers would have to submit pre-market approval applications and present safety and effectiveness data. Then in 1989, when an unpublished study revealed that polyurethane foam in Natural Y breast implants could degrade into a chemical known to cause cancer, the FDA responded by requesting additional information from the manufacturer regarding the chemical makeup and safety testing of polyurethane foam. The manufacturer chose to remove these implants from the market rather than perform the safety testing.

While the controversy surrounding the safety of breast implants raged in corporate boardrooms, the halls of government, medical research journals and the courts, the public remained largely unaware of the controversy until 1990. The horror stories of women with breast implant complications hit the mainstream media when the possible dangers of silicone implants were discussed on a popular news television show, "Face to Face with Connie Chung." Chung interviewed a series of women who traced their symptoms of immune disorders to their implants.[12] Chung's report stirred considerable media interest, and a succession of news articles and reports on the dangers of silicone

---

[12] Chung, Connie. *Face to Face with Connie Chung.* CBS. 05 Dec. 1990.

implants reached the public.

The increase in public awareness resulted in a wave of protests and criticism from women's groups and public health activists. The controversy arose at a time when the American medical profession was already under attack for neglecting the care of women. The National Institute for Health had released a report calling attention to the lack of research dedicated to diseases affecting women and the use of medical devices designed for women that were allegedly produced without adequate testing. In addition, the implant controversy followed on the heels of the Dalkon Shield™ debate, a corporate fiasco in which thousands of women were awarded legal settlements due to injuries they had suffered from a dangerous contraceptive device.

Around the same time, Representative Ted Weiss from New York conducted a congressional hearing dealing with the safety of silicone breast implants. Weiss's investigation revealed that the Dow Corning internal company documents kept secret by the protective court order had never been seen or reviewed by the FDA. Some of these documents showed that Dow's in-house research had established silicone's toxic properties in early studies on animals. After listening to testimony from scientists, physicians, and women who were ill, the congressional hearing report (ultimately issued in 1992) strongly encouraged the FDA to limit the use of breast implants until further research could be completed.[13]

---

[13] United States. Cong. House. Committee on Government Operations. *The FDA's Regulation of Silicone Breast Implants.* 102 Cong., 2nd sess. H. Rept. Dec. 1992. 19 Jan. 2009.

Meanwhile, the lawsuits against manufacturers continued to mount. By this time hundreds of lawsuits had been filed against breast implant manufacturers. In July of 1991, Brenda Toole was awarded $5.4 million in her suit against Baxter, and the following December, the largest award yet, $7.3 million, was given to Marian Hopkins in her case against Dow Corning. Hopkins' attorney leaked several of the "secret" Dow Corning internal documents to a reporter and the documents quickly found their way into the hands of FDA officials who had never seen the documents before. [14]

Within days of reading the documents, FDA Commissioner, David Kessler, called for a voluntary moratorium on the use of silicone gel implants until the advisory panel could review the newly revealed safety information. In February, the FDA Panel reconvened to review additional information on the safety of silicone breast implants and concluded that although there was no established causal link between autoimmune disease and silicone breast implants, they were, nonetheless, recommending that implants only be used only for reconstruction and that women receiving implants participate in scientific protocols. Then in April, the FDA finalized the voluntary moratorium on breast implants and

---

http://www.info-implants.com/BC/0027.html

[14] "Frontline: Breast Implants on Trial: Breast Implant Chronology." *PBS*. 1995-2008. 19 Jan. 2009.

http://www.pbs.org/wgbh/pages/frontline/implants/cron.html

announced the conditions under which silicone implants could be used in clinical studies. The FDA denied applications for silicone gel breast implants for primary augmentations and required that all implant recipients be enrolled in the scientific research protocols.

In February of 1992, Cincinnati attorney Stan Chesley filed a class action lawsuit against Dow Corning. In the same month, Dow Corning replaced its CEO, signaling a change in their approach to the controversy. Under the new CEO, many of the Dow Corning internal memos were released to the public. In March, Dow Corning withdrew from the silicone implant market and set up a fund for further research into the safety of breast implants.[15] They did, however, continue to supply gel to at least one implant manufacturer.

And still, legal cases continued to mount. In December of 1992, Pamela Jean Johnson won $25 million in Johnson versus Bristol-Myers Squibb. By the end of 1993, 12,359 individuals had filed lawsuits against Dow Corning. In March of 1994, a group of breast implant manufacturers settled a class-action lawsuit with Dow Corning as the largest contributor. Other contributors included Baxter, Bristol-Myers Squibb, and 3M. Although manufacturers continued to claim there was no scientific evidence linking silicone breast implants with autoimmune disease, it was,

---

[15] "Frontline: Breast Implants on Trial: Breast Implant Chronology." *PBS*. 1995-2008. 19 Jan. 2009.
http://www.pbs.org/wgbh/pages/frontline/implants/cron.html

nonetheless, the largest class-action settlement in history.[16]

The Saline Controversy

The moratorium enacted by the FDA in 1992 did not explicitly forbid silicone implants. It did, however, require that only mastectomy patients could use them for first-time implantations and that such patients were required participate in research studies. This left only saline implants available to women who wished to have their breasts augmented for cosmetic reasons. Thousands of women opted for this choice as the number of breast implant surgeries increased by 275% between 1992 and 1997.[17]

Saline implants are made with an outer silicone envelope containing a saline solution inside. They were first marketed in the 1960s, but like silicone implants, they were not evaluated for safety until much later. The FDA did not gain the authority to approve medical devices until 1976, and with a backlog of products to evaluate, it was years before they turned their attention to saline filled implants.

Saline implants were believed to be safer than silicone implants because if the envelope ruptured or leaked, only saline fluid would be released into the body. Women who opted for saline implants were subject to the same local complications as those occurring with silicone implants:

---

[16] Ibid.

[17] Krieger, Lloyd M., and William W. Shaw. "The Effect of Increased Consumer Demand on Fees for Aesthetic Surgery: An Economic Analysis." *Plastic and Reconstructive Surgery* 104 (1999): 2312-317.

infection, capsular contracture and rupture or deflation. Also, like their silicone counterparts, saline implants could ripple, harden, change shape or move out of position. Women sometimes reported loss of feeling in the nipple or the breast, and in some cases the implants could also interfere with breast feeding and make the detection of breast cancer more difficult.

Nonetheless, doctors began seeing some of the same symptoms associated with silicone implants in their patients with saline implants. Some women were reporting chronic fatigue, swollen joints, increased number and duration of infections, including viral, bacterial and fungal infections. Symptoms related to immune deficiencies began appearing in women with saline implants.

In January of 1993, the FDA published a proposal in the Federal Register calling for manufacturer's safety and effectiveness data for saline filled implants, and in June of 1994, the agency heard testimony from interested parties. As a result of this testimony, the FDA updated the patient information sheet on the risks of saline implants provided to patients.[18]

The Turning Tide

---

[18] "Timeline of Breast Implant Activities." *FDA Breast Implant Consumer Handbook*. 2004. United States Food and Drug Administration. 16 Aug. 2009: 62-68.
http://www.fda.gov/downloads/MedicalDevices/ProductsandMedicalProc edures/ImplantsandProsthetics/BreastImplants/ucm064263.pdf

Meanwhile, medical research on the problems with both silicone and saline implants continued. Much of it was financed by the companies who were manufacturing and profiting from the industry and then carried out by plastic surgeons who were hardly objective in this matter. In June 1994, *The New England Journal of Medicine* published the Mayo Clinic epidemiology study, which found no increased risk of connective tissue disease in women with silicone implants.[19]

In June of 1995, the same prestigious journal published the "Harvard Nurses Epidemiological Study," which found no increased risk of connective tissue disease in women with silicone implants.[20] By December of 1995, more than twenty studies and abstracts had been published that failed to support a causal relationship between silicone implants and known autoimmune illnesses.[21]

During this time, as well, there was continued controversy in the courts. In May of 1995, Dow Corning filed for bankruptcy under Chapter 11 law, which essentially put a

---

[19] Gabriel, Sherine E., Michael O'Fallon, Leonard T. Kurland, C. Mary Beard, John E. Woods, and Joseph Melton. "Risk of Connective-Tissue Diseases and Other Disorders after Breast Implantation." *The New England Journal of Medicine* 330 (1994): 1697-1702.

[20] Sánchez-Guerrero, Jorge, Graham A. Colditz, Elizabeth W. Carlson, David J. Hunter, Frank E. Speizer, and Matthew H. Liang. "Silicone Breast Implants and the Risk of Connective-Tissue Diseases and Symptoms." *The New England Journal of Medicine* 332 (1995): 1666-670.

[21] "Frontline: Breast Implants on Trial: Breast Implant Chronology." *PBS*. 1995-2008. 19 Jan. 2009.
http://www.pbs.org/wgbh/pages/frontline/implants/cron.html

hold on all litigation against them. By this time 440,000 women had registered in the global settlement against implant manufacturers. Then in October of the same year, Charlotte Mahlum was awarded $13.9 million in a settlement against Dow Chemical, the parent company of Dow Corning. This was the first case in which the parent company of a manufacturer was the sole defendant. In November, a new global settlement was formed with Bristol-Myers Squibb, Baxter and 3M as the participants.[22]

In July of 1998, Dow Corning offered $3.2 billion to settle tens of thousands of claims and the plaintiffs accepted. This agreement allowed Dow Corning to emerge from bankruptcy proceedings. In November of 1998, Dow Corning filed for reorganization under Chapter 11 with a plan that took into effect the $3.2 billion settlement.[23]

Even as manufacturers were settling an enormous number of claims against them, the tide was beginning to change in their favor. Late in 1996, the California Court of Appeals and Oregon Federal Judge Robert Jones had dismissed multiple lawsuits on the basis that scientific studies showed no link to disease. These cases were the first in a series of cases in which manufacturers were able to successfully defend themselves against claims. Their defense was that there was no conclusive evidence in the scientific research that linked implants to systemic disease. Even so, one state court found Dow Chemical guilty of knowingly

---

[22] Ibid.
[23] Ibid.

deceiving women by hiding safety information about silicone.[24]

In 1997, the Department of Health and Human Services asked the Institute of Medicine to conduct an independent review and ongoing scientific research regarding the safety of silicone breast implants. That year, the National Institute of Health hosted a panel workshop to determine whether a link existed between silicone breast implants and atypical rheumatic disease. The NIH panel members generally agreed that based on current data, a link could not be ruled out. The epidemiologists on the panel felt that the current studies were flawed and not large enough to be statistically significant. The panel's findings were reported in the June issue of *Plastic Surgery News*.[25]

In December 1998, a panel of four independent experts were appointed by Judge Samuel C. Pointer, a Federal District Court judge in Birmingham, Alabama, to sift through the conflicting scientific research on the safety of breast implants. The panel concluded that there was no scientific evidence to show that silicone breast implants cause disease. Judge Pointer refused to dismiss the panel's findings after litigants complained that one panel member had taken an honorarium from one of the breast implant manufacturers involved and solicited donations from

---

[24] Ibid.
[25] "NIH Panel Recommends Additional Studies to Investigate Link between Silicone Breast Implants and Atypical Rheumatic Disease." *Plastic Surgery News* June 1997.

another during his tenure on the panel.[26]

In June of 1999, the Institute of Medicine released its comprehensive review of the published literature and ongoing studies entitled "Safety of Silicone Breast Implants."[27] This report concluded that local complications were the primary safety issue with silicone breast implants and there was insufficient evidence to establish that either saline or silicone breast implants caused systemic health effects. The committee did not conduct any original research. They conducted public hearings and examined past research and other materials to come to their conclusion.

In August of 1999, the FDA required manufacturers to submit pre-manufacture applications containing data that would ostensibly establish the relative safety and effectiveness of saline implants. In 2000, the FDA approved pre-manufacture applications from Mentor Corporation and McGhan Corporation for their saline filled breast implants. In the same year, the FDA also approved a proposal from Mentor Corporation for a study of silicone implants for augmentation, reconstruction and revision for a limited number of patients at a limited number of sites.

FDA Re-Approval

In November of 2006, the FDA issued their approval (with

---

[26] "Frontline: Breast Implants on Trial: Breast Implant Chronology." *PBS*.

[27] Unites States. Institute of Medicine. *Safety of Silicone Breast Implants*. Ed. Stuart Bondurant, Virginia Ernster, and Roger Herdman. Washington, DC: National Academy P, 1999.

conditions) to Allergan Corporation (formerly McGhan and Inamed) and Mentor Corporation to market their silicone gel breast implants in the United States. The conditions of the approval required that each company conduct a large post-approval study, continue its studies for ten years, conduct a focus group study of the patient labeling, continue laboratory studies to further characterize types of device failure, and track each implant in the event that health professionals and patients needed to be notified of updated product information.

The American Society of Plastic Surgeons and the American Society for Aesthetic Plastic Surgery launched a joint website, http://www.breastimplantsafety.org, to help with physician and patient education.

After fourteen years of FDA restricted access to the silicone breast implants due to safety concerns, the ban had been lifted. In spite of the health issues hundreds of thousands of women faced as a result of these devices, silicone implants were back on the market. After reviewing the existing literature, the FDA review boards determined that only local complications of the chest wall (such as chronic inflammation, granulomas, and fibrosis) are significant problems associated with silicone gel breast implants, ignoring the experimental, clinical and theoretical proof of systemic illness.

While it is hard to understand how this information could be ignored, it is even more difficult to understand how the FDA could have approved the pre-market applications submitted by Mentor and McGhan when their studies did not follow patients for the length of time required for the

Silastic shell to become incompetent. According to peer-reviewed literature, this lipolytic process takes from eight to fourteen years in most patients,[28,29,30] and the studies submitted to the FDA followed patients for less than five years.[31,32,33]

The other problem with the cohesive gel study is that plastic surgeons were allowed to conduct the research. Patients who participated in the study have reported to me that when they informed the plastic surgeon conducting the study they had developed systemic problems (such as fatigue, muscle aches and mental clouding), they were told their symptoms were not related to their implants. They were told this despite the fact that they also had chest wall symptoms indicating probable infection around the implant. It is likely that these patients were experiencing an infection

---

[28,] Robinson, O. Gordon, Edwin L. Bradley, and Donna S. Wilson. "Analysis of Explanted Silicone Implants: A Report of 300 Patients." *Annals of Plastic Surgery* 34 (1995): 1-6.

[29] Cohen, Benjamin E., Thomas M. Biggs, Ernest D. Cronin, and Donald R. Collins. "Assessment and Longevity of the Silicone Gel Breast Implant." *Plastic and Reconstructive Surgery Journal* 99 (1997): 1697-601.

[30] Pfleiderer, B., T. Campbell, C. A. Hulka, et al. "Silicone Gel-Filled Breast Implants in Women: Findings at H-1 MR Spectroscopy." *Radiology* 201 (1996): 777-83.

[31] US FDA/CDRH. "Breast Implant Questions and Answers (2006)." *U S Food and Drug Administration*. 2006. 10 Feb. 2009.

[32] "Breast Implant Clinical Studies." *Love Your Look*. 2007. Mentor Corporation. 19 Jan. 2009.
http://www.loveyourlook.com/Breast-Implants/clinical-studies.aspx

[33] "Frequently Asked Questions about MemoryGel Implants." *Mentor*. 2007. Mentor Corporation. 19 Jan. 2009.
http://www.memorygel.com/FAQs.aspx

around an implant and possible local inflammation associated with systemic symptoms perhaps mediated by a mold biotoxin or autoimmune reaction to the textured surface of the implant. According to the National Organization of Women, women have reported that they were dropped from the companies' monitoring programs when they became ill. This practice would, of course, have the effect of hiding the health risks of silicone implants.[34]

How long will it take for the corporations who produce breast implants and the government organizations responsible for the regulation of these devices to understand the enormous amount of human suffering that has been created as the result of this situation? I receive phone calls almost daily from women who begin to suffer health problems shortly after receiving implants. Other patients report that they don't have problems until after the Silastic shell begins to break down, which can take a decade. Based on the symptoms patients describe, I suspect that some of these implants may be leaking or leeching chemicals.

Meanwhile, every day hundreds of women undergo augmentation with the new silicone gel implants, and I can only wonder how long the Silastic shell will contain the chemicals or the gel. If we have failed to investigate and understand what happened to the hundreds of thousands of

---

[34] Erickson, Jan. "FDA Bows to Industry: OKs Risky Kind of Breast Implant." National NOW Times. 2007. *National Organization for Women*. 05 Feb. 2009.
http://www.now.org/nnt/winter-2007/breastimplants.html

women who became ill from the silicone gel implants of the 1970s and 1980s, I have little faith that the human recipients of these new "improved" silicone gel implants will have a different destiny. A new generation of women will have to navigate through their unknown illnesses with very little assistance from the medical community.

Joyce's Story

Joyce's story reminds us that many patients who win the battle with breast cancer succumb to a serious, debilitating disease from chemical and silicone toxicity from their breast implant reconstructions. Her story shows us the extent to which the medical profession ignores this disease, even though reports of fibromyalgia and other problems secondary to ruptured silicone breast implants are abundant in the medical literature. Joyce emphasizes a woman's right to know in order to make an informed decision. Her story also demonstrates the importance of taking charge of your own recovery. Joyce trusted her own judgment, rather than following medical advice that did not make sense to her. Because she took responsibility for discovering the source of her illness, she is alive today.

"It had been eighteen years since I lost both my breasts to cancer. I was 42 years old at the time and there was no question that I would have reconstructive surgery. I had complete confidence in my surgeon and plastic surgeon.

There was a brief discussion about the various options, but there was no doubt in their minds that silicone implants were preferable for getting the most natural look.

"I elected to have the reconstruction immediately and expanders were placed under my chest wall at the time my diseased breasts were removed. The following months of stretching my chest muscles so that they would accommodate the implants while I received chemotherapy were painfully difficult. The physical pain was acute and the emotional pain of losing my breasts and fearing death from cancer were overwhelming at times. If it had not been for the tender loving care of my family and friends, I am afraid I would have become unbearably depressed and discouraged.

"At last, the day came for the final surgery and the silicone implants were permanently placed under my chest wall. Again, there was more pain and more emotional upheaval as I adjusted to more pain and healing and, of course, there was my new look. While I was pleased with the results of the reconstructive surgery, and my plastic surgeon was considered one of the best in the nation (some say that he literally "wrote the book" on breast reconstruction), it was still a terribly difficult emotional adjustment. I was still a young women and my whole body image had changed.

"So many emotions and issues, not the least was the battle with cancer, happened during that time that it never occurred to me to ask many questions about the silicone implants I received. No one offered any specific information about the implants. I hadn't heard about any dangers related to the silicone or been told anything about the fact that they would inevitably deteriorate and need to be replaced.

"Less then a year later, the news was full of claims that implants made women ill and caused many disturbing symptoms and conditions. Of course, I asked my physicians about all this and was reassured that it was all a tempest in a teacup and there was no "science" to support any negative claims. I trusted my doctors. I also decided to put the whole matter out my mind and focus on staying healthy and cancer free. That seemed like the bigger issue, even when the FDA took the silicone implants off the market.

"I did stay amazingly healthy. I made health and wellness a major focus of my life and managed to stay cancer free for the next 18 years. Then I started getting sick. I was also fatigued to the point of tears on a daily basis. I lived for the weekends when I could sleep. I owned my own business, which had taken huge personal energy over a fifteen-year period. That energy had always been there and now it was gone. I began complaining about this debilitating fatigue to my doctors.

"They ran tests and more tests. Nothing accounted for the chronic fatigue or the multiple bouts of bronchitis, colds, allergies and other ailments. I had rarely been sick in the previous fifteen years. More than one doctor was patronizing and would agree to check out some other medical possibility after I insisted.

"Of course, I was afraid of a cancer recurrence, but my intuitive feeling was that the fatigue and immune system malfunction, which is what I called my condition, was not cancer. By now, I was also experiencing some anxiety and depression because I was self-employed, and self-employed people do not have sick leave. No work means no pay. Not only that, I had a private practice in psychotherapy. I worked with children and adolescents and their families and many people counted on me being there and being able to help them.

"Then, a good thing happened. I found a lump in my right breast. At no time in the previous eighteen years did I ever consider a breast lump to be a good thing. Actually, I didn't this time. I did know that something had to be done immediately. A couple months prior to finding the lump, I had consulted a plastic surgeon (my original surgeon had passed away) about getting my nipples re-tattooed. The original tattoos had faded, and I wanted to get them redone. At that time, the doctor mentioned that my implants were quite old, and they probably should be "checked." However, there were only one or two places that had the necessary MRI equipment, and those places were over an hour away. It just did not seem like a necessary test.

"This doctor did not mention silicone poisoning, symptoms related to silicone leakage and, most especially, silicone traveling to my lymph nodes. He never even suggested that there might be some urgency or danger related to not investigating further. He did say that the implants were never designed to last so many years. This was the first time I had ever heard such a thing. Still, there was no outward sign that my implants were collapsed or leaking, and I did not pursue the matter further---until I found the lump.

"When I found the lump, I immediately went to see the surgeon that did my original mastectomies. She ordered an ultrasound and an MRI. When the results came, there was evidence that at least one of the implants was leaking but the surgeon said that leaking implants were to be expected and surely did not warrant concern. After all, she explained that my body had long ago formed a natural capsule around the implants, so there was no reason to suspect that the silicone was outside those natural capsules. She said that I should be careful not to get hit in the chest, but other than that, I should not worry. If I was determined to pursue the matter, she would refer me to a plastic surgeon.

"She again asserted that there was no "science" behind any of the accusations about silicone poisoning, and if I wanted to go to the extreme of having the implants removed, she would consider it a waste at best, and foolish at the least. I had trusted this woman with my very survival. I respected her. I wanted to believe her but what she said, especially about trying to be sure not to "poke around" in my breast and not let myself get hit, just did not make sense to me. It didn't make common sense.

"Finally, I decided to seek a second opinion from a plastic surgeon that was not associated with my surgeon. I remembered a woman I had met some years before who had had breast cancer and many years later had experienced serious medical problems that could not be defined. I still made no connection with my battle with fatigue or repeated infections with my "could be leaking" implants. I just recalled that this woman had issues with her implants. I called her and she referred me to Dr. Susan Kolb.

"By the time I reached Dr. Kolb, I had already had several ultrasounds, an MRI and every other blood test, chest x-ray and heart stress test that could possibly be ordered. I will never forget Dr. Kolb's first comments to me after reviewing the ultrasound and MRI results. "You must be experiencing extreme fatigue," she said, and then went on to describe the many medical problems I had been having in the past several years.

"She assured me that the silicone was indeed dangerous to my health and that the implants would eventually be removed from the market again. She showed me the research on silicone poisoning. She said that it was sad that no one, not the surgeon, the plastic surgeon, my primary care physician, my gynecologist or any doctor that I had seen in the last several years had ever suggested to me that my silicone implants could be the cause of my recent medical problems.

"To me it was more than sad. It was outrageous. How could this be? Every doctor I had seen knew that I had had cancer and that I had implants. None ever suggested that there could be any problem related to the implants. If Dr. Kolb was right about my symptoms, then clearly work had to be done to alert every woman with silicone implants about the dangers to their health. Two weeks after my initial visit with Dr. Kolb, I had the explant surgery. It took eight hours to get all the silicone that had seeped out of the implants. Silicone was found in my lymph glands. Clearly the silicone was in other areas of my body. I began a long, slow, painful recovery.

"It was unbearably hard to have my breasts removed the first time. The explant operation felt like déjà vu. It did not seem possible that I was going through all of this again. I had come to accept my silicone breasts and felt that they looked pretty good. Now I was back to fears of yet another body image adjustment, not to mention fear of what the lump, which drove me to the surgeon's office in the first place, might be. Most of all, I had to recover my health. I found it more difficult at age sixty than age forty-two.

"Dr. Kolb's after surgery care was even more meticulous than the excellent surgery that she performed. This time the lump was benign. The new saline implants looked better than ever, and best of all, three months after the painful and traumatic surgery, I experienced a return of my physical energy. It was like finding out that a friend I thought was dead was found alive. Friends and family kept commenting about how good I looked, and I felt great. It was amazing and wonderfully exciting.

"I have to admit that it had been easy for me to believe that my silicone implants should be removed. Once I knew they were leaking, common sense demanded their removal. It had been harder for me to believe that the leaking silicone could be the cause of my chronic fatigue, chronic infections and other problematic symptoms. But there could be no mistake. Every day I feel the positive changes in my body and most of all my renewed energy.

"Now I want to use some of that energy to educate physicians and women everywhere who have, or are considering having, silicone implants about the risks and facts related to silicone. The least these women deserve is the ability to make an informed decision. They deserve to be told that silicone implants need to be replaced every eight years before they have a chance to deteriorate, and they deserve to be told the facts about the potential of silicone poisoning.

"If we are given warnings about every other medical

intervention including aspirin, why not silicone implants? How could giving this information be harmful to anyone except possibly the manufacturers of the implants? Women have a right to know. I wish I had known.

-3-
SILICONE IMMUNE DISEASE

"Two things are infinite: The universe and human stupidity; and I'm not sure about the universe."
Albert Einstein

Silicone Immune Disease can occur when silicone gel leaks outside the Silastic shell of breast implants. The disorder stems from the effects of free silicone, as well as the chemicals used in the manufacturing process, acting on the various systems of the body. Patients can present more than twenty symptoms, many of them vague, like muscle aches, chronic fatigue and brain fog. The illness progresses slowly over a number of years and can be difficult to diagnose. Nonspecific diagnoses of arthritis, chronic fatigue syndrome and fibromyalgia are common. Women often don't connect their symptoms with their implants and even if they do, their physicians may tell them their implants cannot possibly be causing their illnesses.

Once the silicone gel leaks out of the Silastic shell, either as a result of the body's lipolysis reaction (the attempt to break down the implant casing, gradually weakening the shell and allowing the silicone to slowly seep out) or to an actual rupture of the shell, the problems caused by free silicone in a woman's body are obviously not limited to the chest wall, even though implant companies and plastic surgeons often tell her they are. When the silicone leaks from the casing, it migrates throughout the body, affecting every organ and system of the body. As early as 1956, researchers at Dow Chemical had established that liquid silicone injected into animals migrated to all the major organs and affected the brain, heart, lungs and spleen.

In 1970, research at both Dow Corning and Dow Chemical again confirmed that silicone migrates to all parts of the body, finding evidence of silicone in bone marrow and noting a reduction in brain weight in the animals they studied.[1] In 1998, research scientists at Baylor College of Medicine found that silicone injected into mice migrated to ten different organs.[2] In 1999, researchers reported that

---

[1] Kennedy, Ron. "Silicone Implant Disease." *The Doctors' Medical Library.* 15 Jan. 1999. 01 Feb. 2009.
http://www.medical-library.net/content/view/91/41/
[2] Kala, Subbarao V., Ernest D. Lykissa, Matthew W. Neely, and Michael W. Lieberman. "Low Molecular Weight Silicones Are Widely Distributed after a Single Subcutaneous Injection in Mice." *American Journal of Pathology* 152 (1998): 645-49.

silicone injections in mice resulted in fatal liver and lung damage.[3]

When breast implants rupture or leak, the silicone released into the human body has the same effect as silicone injections. According to professors at the University of Tennessee, "There is little if any difference between the effects of direct injections of silicone and the effects of gel-filled devices (implants)."[4] A number of studies have shown that silicone implants are likely to leak within ten years of surgical placement, releasing free silicone into the body.[5,6,7] In 1995, FDA Commissioner David Kessler estimated that the rupture rate of silicone implants ranges between 5% and 51%.[8] Dr. Lu-Jean Feng, a plastic surgeon at Mt. Sinai Medical Center, presented evidence to the Plaintiff's Steering Committee for the National Breast Implant

---

[3] Lieberman, Michael William, Ernest D. Lykissa, Roberto Barrios, Ching Nan Ou, Geeta Kala, and Subbarao V. Kala. "Cyclosiloxanes Produce Fatal Liver and Lung Damage in Mice." *Environmental Health Perspectives* 107 (1999): 161-65.

[4] Leviton, Richard, "Poisoned Breasts." *Alternative Medicine* (Nov. 1998): 48-54.

[5] Robinson, O. Gordon, Edwin L. Bradley, and Donna S. Wilson. "Analysis of Explanted Silicone Implants: A Report of 300 Patients." *Annals of Plastic Surgery* 34 (1995): 1-6.

[6] Cohen, Benjamin E., Thomas M. Biggs, Ernest D. Cronin, and Donald R. Collins. "Assessment and Longevity of the Silicone Gel Breast Implant." *Plastic and Reconstructive Surgery Journal* 99 (1997): 1697-601.

[7] Pfleiderer, B., T. Campbell, C. A. Hulka, et al.. "Silicone Gel-Filled Breast Implants in Women: Findings at H-1 MR Spectroscopy." *Radiology* 201 (1996): 777-83.

[8] Leviton, Richard, "Poisoned Breasts." *Alternative Medicine* (Nov. 1998): 48-54.

Litigation which indicated that the rupture rate of implants which have been in the body for less than seven years is 11%, while the rupture rate of implants in the body for longer than seven years is 61%. [9]

From the study of the literature, we have learned that scavenger cells called macrophages pick up the free silicone and carry it into the lymphatic system where it gains access to the rest of the body. The silicone and chemicals in the gel are toxic to the macrophages, and digestion of these materials by the macrophages is not possible. Therefore, the macrophages discharge the material elsewhere in the body where it is picked up by other macrophages.

This process leads to an increase in the release of cytokines or inflammatory intermediates, which promote local inflammation and pain. This is why I experienced, as did most of my patients, a burning sensation in the tissues around the leaking implant when the Silastic shell of the implant was no longer functioning to keep the silicone gel and the associated chemicals inside the shell. This burning in my chest wall gradually increased and eventually affected my left arm, as that was the side on which my implant was leaking. Some women experience a burning sensation equally on both sides of their chest with the sensation traveling down their arm as their illness progresses.

The Department of Radiology Sciences at UCLA published an abstract entitled "Compromising

---

[9] Leviton, Richard, "Poisoned Breasts." *Alternative Medicine* (Nov. 1998): 48-54.

Abnormalities of the Brachial Plexus as Displayed by Magnetic Resonance Imaging" by Collins, Shaver, Disher and Miller[10]. When I read the article, it became clear to me why I had increasing neurological problems with my left arm. Nerve conduction testing and a neurological exam later confirmed the diagnosis as thoracic outlet syndrome, as well as conduction delays along the median nerve associated with sensory and motor deficits.

Fortunately, I am right handed, and other than experiencing numbness of my left upper extremity (usually at night after lying on my left side), this disability did not affect my functioning (except to prevent me from performing certain yoga postures) and had no effect on my ability to perform surgery. Some of my patients, especially those with ruptured implants, had much more severe neurological problems.

Because of the dysfunction of the lymphatic drainage of the arm when silicone clogs up the lymphatic channels in the axilla, many patients experienced swelling of the extremities, and many underwent carpal tunnel release as the median nerve became entrapped at the wrist due to this swelling. Unfortunately, some women also had an entrapment due to the silicone around the brachial plexus (large nerves) in their axilla (armpit), and when the median nerve scarred to the tissues near the wrist after the carpal

---

[10] Collins, James D., Marla L. Shaver, Anthony C. Disher, and Theodore Q. Miller. "Compromising Abnormalities of the Brachial Plexus as Displayed by Magnetic Resonance Imaging." *Clinical Anatomy* 8 (1995): 1-16.

tunnel surgery, they experienced neurological problems when they extended their arm, due to stretching of the nerves between these two fixed points.

Silicone Disease and Surgery

It became clear to me that surgical removal of the silicone was mostly achieved only in the chest wall and in the lymph nodes closest to the chest wall where most of the silicone was entrapped. Removal of these larger infected and inflamed lymph nodes was advisable, especially as I realized that the majority of breast implant patients dying in my practice were dying of lymphoma.

Chemicals in the silicone gel that had reached these lymph nodes were known to be carcinogens as well as neurotoxins. Concern about anaplastic large-cell lymphoma developing in this patient population had been expressed in a communication to JAMA in November of 2008[11].

Although it was not advisable to remove multiple lymph nodes, especially if they were not enlarged or firm, I found clinically that removing the abnormal lymph nodes aided in the recovery of neurological function on the side from which the lymph nodes were removed. I also hoped that the

---

[11] de Jong, Daphne, Wies L. E. Varmel, Jan Paul de Boer, Gideon Verhave, Ellis Barbé, Mariel Casparie and Flora E. van Leeuwen. "Anaplastic Large-Cell Lymphoma in Women with Breast Implants." *Journal of the American Medical Association.* 2008; 300: 2030-2035.

removal of lymph nodes would decrease the rate of lymphoma developing in this patient population.

In order to remove the majority of the silicone gel in the chest wall without spilling the contents of the implants into the breast or chest wall, I routinely remove the scar capsule surrounding the implant in one piece or "en bloc." This helps prevent the escape of the silicone gel, which can be either firm or runny, but in either case is difficult to remove from the tissues once it has escaped the capsule. In the early 1990s, plastic surgeons were not routinely removing the scar capsules, as there was a misconception that the scar capsule would dissolve once the implant was removed.

Pathological examination of the capsules showed foreign body granulomatous reaction, a response to the silicone within the scar capsule. In this type of reaction, the body recognizes the silicone as "not self," walls it off with scar tissue and surrounds it with inflammatory cells. Later, articles in the plastic surgery literature indicated that if the capsules were not removed, there was a greater risk of postoperative complications including infection and fluid collections called seromas.[12]

In some cases, the silicone gel had already traveled beyond the capsule and was forming granulomas or hard tender nodules within the muscles or the breast tissue. In one case, I had to remove the majority of the pectoralis chest

---

[12] Hardt, N. S., L. Yu, G. LaTorre, and B. Steinbach. "Complications Related to Retained Breast Implant Capsules." *Plastic and Reconstructive Surgery Journal* 95 (1995): 364-71.

wall muscle due to involvement of the muscle with a large silicone granuloma. This patient had a markedly elevated CPK level (an abnormally high level of the enzyme creatinine kinase) indicating muscle damage.

After removal of this silicone granuloma from the muscle, these lab values returned to normal. I had a conversation with the patient's rheumatologist who did not believe that silicone caused autoimmune disease, but had to admit in this case that the silicone granuloma was related to the abnormal lab test.

Many patients have had the release of the pectoralis muscle insertion during the surgery to place the implants, especially if large implants were inserted. It is important to reattach these muscle insertions if possible in order to avoid chest wall deformities. Patients with multiple surgeries are especially at risk for removal of the chest wall muscles, either because these are incorporated with the capsule or because surgeons who do not realize how difficult the dissection is between the capsule and the chest wall muscles remove them inadvertently.

If a surgeon tells a patient that he or she is able to remove the implants and capsules in one to two hours, the surgeon is likely speaking from inexperience. The more tissue removed, the more likely the patient is to have a permanent chest wall deformity. Tissue that is incorporated in the capsule or within a silicone granuloma must be removed in order to avoid post-operative problems.

Explantation surgery is much more difficult than implantation, so it is important to find a qualified surgeon. If a surgeon does not believe implants are associated with health problems, he or she is less likely to spend the time necessary to remove the entire capsule. Retained capsules are associated with problems such as seroma formation, infection and problems with imaging for cancer screening in the future.

Chemical Soup

Further evaluation of the chemical makeup of silicone gel may explain why systemic illness can occur after it leaks into the body. According to *Truth about Implants*, a group providing support for women affected by breast implants, information reported from the manufacturers and the court documents indicate that thirty-seven chemicals are used in making silicone implant gel.[13] The group's website lists the following chemicals as ingredients:

1. Methyl ethyl ketone (neurotoxin)
2. Cyclohexanone (neurotoxin)
3. Isopropyl alcohol
4. Denatured alcohol
5. Acetone (neurotoxin)

---

[13] "Chemical Composition of Breast Implants." *Truth About Implants*. 2008. 19 Jan. 2009. http://www.truthaboutbreastimplants.com/get_sick.html

6. Urethane
7. Polyvinyl chloride (neurotoxin)
8. Amine
9. Toluene (neurotoxin/carcinogen)
10. Dichloromethane (carcinogen)
11. Chloromethane
12. Ethyl acetate (neurotoxin)
13. Silicone
14. Sodium fluoride
15. Lead-based solder
16. Formaldehyde
17. Talcum powder
18. Oakite (cleaning solvent)
19. Methyl 2-cyanoacrylates
20. Ethylene oxide (carcinogen)
21. Xylene (neurotoxin)
22. Hexon
23. 2-Hexanone
24. Thixon-OSN-2
25. Stearic acid
26. Zinc oxide
27. Naptha (rubber solvent)
28. Phenol (neurotoxin)
29. Benzene (carcinogen/neurotoxin)
30. Lacquer thinner
31. Epoxy resin
32. Epoxy hardener 10 and 11
33. Printing ink
34. Metal cleaning acid
35. Color pigments as release agents
36. Heavy metals such as aluminum and platinum
37. Silica

Any plastic surgeon reviewing this list of chemicals should be able to understand why after approximately eight to ten years, silicone patients may present with symptoms of a progressive illness with features of immune, neurological and endocrine problems. Indeed, despite the Institute of Medicine's conclusion that "There was insufficient evidence to establish that either or both types of breast implants cause systemic health effects, such as autoimmune disease,"[14] Douglas R. Shanklin, M.D., professor of pathology and of obstetrics and gynecology at the University of Tennessee in Memphis, believes that there is a relationship. His extensive research involving implant patients demonstrates that "immune processing and inflammatory cell responses are commonplace in the tissues surrounding silicone mammary implants."[15] Dr. Shanklin concludes that the cellular conditions he has observed can be attributed to a new form of autoimmunity. He reports:

> It has now been confirmed that: 1) silicone induces atypical antibodies and peptides through changes in native tissue proteins, 2) there is clear-cut cellular immunity, lymphocytes and macrophages, principal means by which the body responds to silicone and silica, a major device component and silicone breakdown products, 3) the lymphocyte stimulation involves interleukin-2, part of the system of chemical signals between inflammatory cells, and

---

[14] "Timeline of Breast Implant Activities." *FDA Breast Implant Consumer Handbook*. 2004. United States Food and Drug Administration. 19 Jan. 2009: 62-68.
http://www.fda.gov/downloads/MedicalDevices/ProductsandMedicalProcedures/ImplantsandProsthetics/BreastImplants/ucm064263.pdf
[15] Shanklin, Douglas R. and David L. Smalley. "Quantitative Aspects of Cellular Responses to Silicone." *International Journal of Occupational Medicine and Toxicology* 4 (1995): 99-111.

there is growing evidence of progression into plasma cell myeloma, an unusual malignancy of the immune system and certain precursor disorders.[16]

Sadly, evidence has now begun to accumulate that children born after a woman has these devices implanted are likely to be in poor health. The children show lymphocyte sensitization indices at about half the maternal levels, indicating an impaired immune system. Children born to the same women before they received implants had normal health and showed normal growth and development.

Dr. Shanklin once told me that his best chemical analysis of the breast implants was that they were "a bag full of silicone garbage." Since it is well known that chemicals can trigger autoimmune disease, it should not be a surprise to anyone that once these chemicals leak into the body, an autoimmune disease results.

Any physician who has studied the patient population at risk has seen a variety of autoimmune problems, the majority of which do not fall into any known disease category. Some patients have symptoms similar to patients with scleroderma, rheumatoid arthritis, lupus, and multiple sclerosis, *but* the most common diagnosis these women receive from competent physicians is atypical connective tissue disease and atypical neurological disease.

It becomes clear why the early epidemiological studies

---

[16] Shanklin, Douglas R. "Article by Dr. Douglas R. Shanklin." *Info-Implants.* 1996. 19 Jan. 2009
http://www.info-implants.com/Walt/172.html

done at Harvard, Duke, and Mayo clinic failed to show a correlation between known autoimmune diseases and silicone gel implants. *It is not possible to perform an epidemiological study on a disease that has not yet been characterized.* While it is true that silicone breast implants do not cause the autoimmune diseases listed in these studies, it is not true that they are not the root cause of the patients' symptoms. Since these patients do not have scleroderma, rheumatoid arthritis, lupus or multiple sclerosis, it is not difficult to show a lack of correlation between their symptoms and these illnesses. Instead, these patients are suffering from silicone immune disease, a new illness that has not been identified or characterized and for which laboratory tests confirming their diagnosis do not yet exist. Instead of using science to develop and treat their conditions, medical science is being used in the service of corporate interests to disprove their conditions.

The Ethical Irony

It is a common practice for the institutions conducting the research into the safety of breast implants to receive endowments from Dow Corning, Dow Chemical or other interested corporate concerns. This practice, in and of itself, can be considered a conflict of interest and raises questions about the possibility of scientific bias in the research.

In the early part of 2000, I interviewed Dr. Andrew Campbell on my radio show. Dr. Campbell was one of the editors of *The International Journal of Occupational Medicine and Toxicology*'s 1995 special issue on silicone toxicology.[17] He told the story of a professor of urology at a famous medical clinic, who after announcing a proposed study on the systemic effects of penile implants (which are made of silicone), lost his position and was replaced. It should not come as a surprise that very few studies on the toxicology of silicone come out of the institutions that are endowed by the chemical industry's deep pockets.

Even the federal government, including the FDA and Institute of Medicine (a part of the National Institute of Health), are heavily influenced by the corporations involved in the manufacturing of the very products under consideration. Much of the research that has been done in this area has been done by the research and development divisions of the corporations themselves or in academic or medical research facilities endowed by the same corporations.

The corporate influence is so substantial that the FDA even ignored clinical research published in a peer-reviewed journal that they had partially funded. The research, published in *The Journal of Rheumatology*, showed that women with ruptured implants had an increased incidence of fibromyalgia, a disease known to be associated with

---

[17] Brautbar, Nachman, Andrew Campbell, and Aristo Vojdani, eds. *International Journal of Occupational Medicine and Toxicology.* Special Issue on Silicone Toxicity. 4 (1995).

chemical toxicity.[18] In spite of this, the FDA approved silicone implants for sale to consumers.

In 2005, FDA Commissioner, Lester Crawford resigned when it was discovered that he owned stocks in food, beverage and medical device companies he was in charge of regulating. He later pleaded guilty to conflict of interest and falsely reporting information.[19] In approving silicone breast implants for sale, the FDA ignored information provided by three company whistle blowers who alleged that Mentor had "falsified data, failed to disclose damaging information about leaky valves and rupture rates and — most alarmingly — failed to report accurate information about levels of a form of oxidized platinum in the implants that is known to be harmful to humans. In all three cases, the FDA did not require new studies to evaluate the allegations." [20]

In November 2008, FDA scientists wrote a letter to Congress accusing top officials in the agency of approving unsafe medical devices. The letter claims that research scientists were ordered to change their opinions and

[18] Brown, S., G. Pennello, and M. Soo. "Silicone Gel Breast Implant Rupture, Extracapsular Silicone and Health Status in a Population of Women." *Journal of Rheumatology* 28 (2001): 996-1003.
[19] "Implants and the FDA." *HADCORP: Knowledge Empowers.* Human Adjuvant Disease Corp. 02 Feb. 2009.
http://implants.webs.com/implantsandthefda.htm
[20] Erickson, Jan. "FDA Bows to Industry: OKs Risky Kind of Breast Implant." *National NOW Times.* 2007. National Organization for Women. 05 Feb. 2009.
http://www.now.org/nnt/winter-2007/breastimplants.html

conclusions to expedite FDA approval of medical devices.[21] These are only a few examples that demonstrate the disturbing degree of conflict of interest between the FDA and the companies they are charged with regulating. Unfortunately, corporate interests cannot be trusted to serve public health.

The Plastic Surgeon's Dilemma

I have described my clinical findings regarding silicone, chemical and biotoxicity to a number of my plastic surgery colleagues. There are a few, mostly hand surgeons who do not perform many breast augmentation procedures, who grasp the significance of what I've found clinically. The majority of the plastic surgeons who perform silicone breast reconstruction and augmentation, however, respond in a much different manner to this information. Most are fairly incredulous and change the subject, as it is quite uncomfortable for them to consider.

Certainly most physicians think of themselves as moral and reasonable people. It is much more comfortable to believe that which has been quoted on the evening news than to actually review the medical literature on the subject, especially when what is on the evening news is what they want to believe. The problem is that a part of them knows that what I'm saying is true, for the women who are chronically ill have come to them, and some of these women even received their silicone breast implants from these

---

[21] Harris, Gardiner. "F.D.A. Scientists Accuse Agency Officials of Misconduct." *The New York Times* [New York] 18 Nov. 2008. 19 Jan, 2009 http://www.nytimes.com/2008/11/18/health/policy/18fda.html

surgeons.

It is easy to say that there is no scientific research that supports systemic problems with silicone breast implants. It is easy to say that saline implants are safe. The problem with these statements is that they are simply not true. Indeed, the chronically ill women they see before them, sitting in their offices, provide the most convincing evidence available.

These plastic surgeons may now feel vindicated in their position because the FDA has returned silicone gel implants to that market. However, the scientific studies that the FDA reviewed only followed women with breast implants for three years after implantation (Mentor) and four years (Allergan).[22,23,24] Some, of the women in these studies have contacted me to report that when they told their plastic surgeons they were having systemic symptoms, the surgeons told them that their implants were not causing these problems. The National Organization of Women also heard reports that women who complained of systemic symptoms

---

[22] US FDA. "Breast Implant Questions and Answers (2006)." *U S Food and Drug Administration.* 2006. 10 Feb. 2009.
http://www.fda.gov/cdrh/breastimplants/qa2006.html#s2
[23] "Frequently Asked Questions about MemoryGel Implants." *Mentor.* 2007. Mentor Corporation. 19 Jan. 2009.
http://www.memorygel.com/FAQs.aspx
[24] "Breast Implant Clinical Studies." *Love Your Look.* 2007. Mentor Corporation. 19 Jan. 2009.
http://www.loveyourlook.com/Breast-Implants/clinical-studies.aspx

were eliminated from the companies' studies.[25] Therefore I find it likely that the studies were not entirely unbiased. The scientific data indicates that the shell starts to break down eight to ten years after implantation,[26,27,28] so any study that does not follow the women's health for more than ten years is seriously flawed.

Of course the real difficulty in these studies lies in their design. Scientific studies can be designed to produce a desired outcome, and when research is conducted by corporate research departments or agencies funded by corporations with a vested interest in the study's outcome, it is impossible to discount the possibility of bias.

Some doctors and scientists also contend that since epidemiological studies have not conclusively established a link between silicone breast implants and autoimmune disease that the implants are therefore safe. They argue that the "scientific" evidence is not sufficient to establish a cause-effect relationship because of the insufficiency of

---

[25] Erickson, Jan. "FDA Bows to Industry: OKs Risky Kind of Breast Implant." *National NOW Times.* 2007. National Organization for Women. 05 Feb. 2009.
http://www.now.org/nnt/winter-2007/breastimplants.html
[26] Robinson, O. Gordon, Edwin L. Bradley, and Donna S. Wilson. "Analysis of Explanted Silicone Implants: A Report of 300 Patients." *Annals of Plastic Surgery* 34 (1995): 1-6.
[27] Cohen, Benjamin E., Thomas M. Biggs, Ernest D. Cronin, and Donald R. Collins. "Assessment and Longevity of the Silicone Gel Breast Implant." *Plastic and Reconstructive Surgery Journal* 99 (1997): 1697-601.
[28] Pfleiderer, B., T. Campbell, C. A. Hulka, et al. "Silicone Gel-Filled Breast Implants in Women: Findings at H-1 MR Spectroscopy." *Radiology* 201 (1996): 777-83.

epidemiological data. However, as David S. Egilman, M.D., clinical associate professor at Brown University School of Medicine, argues in his article "Breast Implants and Disease," the scientific community has never relied solely upon epidemiology as the method of evaluating cause-effect relations in making medical decisions.[29] He writes,

> In making such judgments regarding medical causation, doctors utilize epidemiological data as one tool among many. Although doctors consider epidemiological research to be an important facet of medical epistemology, it is not regarded as being the sole or the most important contributor to decision-making. The branch of medical science concerned with the causes and origins of disease is called etiology. Epidemiology is not a synonym for etiology. Rather, etiologists use epidemiological evidence along with other evidence to draw conclusions about causal connections. Medical knowledge is based on empirical tests. Empirical tests are those gained from observation or experience. [3] Epidemiology is but one form of empirical knowledge.[30]

Egilman cites observation, experiment, analogy, computer models, animal experiments and bacteriologic experiments, as well as epidemiological studies, as the kinds of data doctors consider in establishing a causal relationship. He claims it is not reasonable to ignore entire

---

[29] Egilman, David S. "Breast Implants and Disease." *Info Implants*. 1992. 19 Jan. 2008
http://www.info-implants.com/Blais
[30] Egilman.

classes of data or to elevate one class of data and make sound medical decisions, especially those involving public policy regarding potential health risks.

According to Egilman, most doctors who treat patients rely more on clinical data to make decisions regarding diagnosis, especially in cases involving occupational and environmental diseases. In fact, the patient's history is the most important piece of information in determining if a disease or injury is related to exposure.[31]

Yet in the controversy over the safety of breast implants, epidemiological studies have been elevated over other types of empirical data, and viewed by the FDA and the medical community as "carrying the ultimate burden of proof." Egilman invokes the history of the tobacco industry's effort to "disprove" the dangers of smoking to make his point:

...scientists working for tobacco companies argued that cigarettes had not been proven to cause lung cancer because of the lack of animal studies establishing such a relationship, because the exact mechanism of cancer induction is unknown and the specific carcinogenic substance(s) is (are) unknown.[32]

Our observation of smokers over long periods of time, however, demonstrates quite a different outcome, and today virtually no one argues that there is no link between smoking and lung cancer. Egilman clearly sees the implant

---

[31] Egilman.
[32] Egilman.

manufacturers' emphasis on epidemiological studies as a calculated maneuver to protect them from financial liability. He writes:

> Prior to the onset of litigation related to silicone breast implants (SBI), manufacturers never suggested that epidemiologic studies were necessary to determine the relationship of any health problem to SBI. SBI manufacturers never conducted, proposed nor sponsored any epidemiologic study of any known problem associated with SBI including contracture, migration, infection, hematoma, or rheumatologic complaint. The manufacturer's lack of interest in following the health effects of their products in women with epidemiological surveillance is further demonstrated by their failure to establish a registry of users or a systematic complaint mechanism for users.[33]

The irony here is that science, a field of endeavor designed to systematically uncover to the truth, has been used to sabotage the truth in the service of corporate survival.

Perhaps one of the most glaring examples of the ethical dilemma surrounding the breast implant controversy occurred inside the ranks of Dow Corning Corporation. In the book, *Informed Consent*, a journalist chronicles the story of John Swanson, the executive who created and supervised Dow's ethics program. Swanson's wife, Colleen, had breast implants, and over the ensuing seventeen-year

---

[33] Egilman.

period, she developed a progression of debilitating symptoms, including migraines, joint and back pain, numbness in her hands and feet and extreme fatigue. Swanson found himself in a personal ethical crisis and ultimately asked to be recused from any connection with Dow's implant business. Colleen had her implants removed in 1991 and filed a lawsuit against her husband's employer. The lawsuit was settled in 1993, the same year Swanson, after being ostracized at work, retired.[34]

In 2004, the Ethics Committee of the American Society of Plastic Surgeons contacted me. They had received a complaint from a local plastic surgeon alleging that I was unnecessarily removing breast implants and practicing surgery without a scientific basis. After speaking with one of the members of the committee at length about both silicone and saline breast implant problems and providing the committee with a large stack of scientific articles defending the basis of my practice, all the charges were dropped, except one.

The committee had reviewed my website and read my article "Doctor, Are You Listening?"[35] They requested I make several changes, including the removal of a reference comparing the toxic effects of silicone poisoning to the

---

[34] Byrne, John A. *Informed Consent*. New York: McGraw-Hill, 1995.
[35] Kolb, Susan E. "Doctor, Are You Listening?" 1996. *Millennium Healthcare*. 19 Jan. 2009.
http://plastikos.com/documents/DoctorAreYouListeningTheSiliconeCatas trophe.pdf

effects of arsenic poisoning. In a letter I received from the chair of the committee, he referred to the article as my "marketing material" and explained the committee's concern that the article contained misleading statements, which might "appeal to a lay person's fears, anxieties or emotional vulnerabilities." While I complied with the Committee's request, I took the opportunity to update the information and include references to the peer-reviewed literature. My arguments were strengthened considerably by the revision. What strengthens my arguments more than anything else is that my patients get better.

The Silicone Immune Protocol

As meticulous as our efforts were during surgery, I knew we were not removing all the silicone gel or chemicals from the chest wall and lower axilla, and I knew that silicone and chemicals had traveled outside the operative field. Articles in the plastic surgery literature indicated that the longer the patient waited before explantation, the less likely they were to recover their health.[36]

I had a unique opportunity, as well as personal inspiration (as a great deal of silicone had been left in my chest wall by my surgeons), to develop an alternative method of removing the silicone from my body. I set about

---

[36] Brawer, A. "Chronology of Systemic Disease Development in 300 Symptomatic Recipients of Silicone Gel-Filled Breast Implants." *Journal of Clean Technology* 5 (1996): 223-33.

this process by studying detoxification protocols in holistic medicine. I began an extensive research process and read everything I could find in the literature. In the late 1990s, I was invited to host an hour-long weekly radio show on holistic medicine on a local Atlanta station. Hosting this program, which later evolved into *The Temple of Health* radio show, gave me the opportunity to interview authors and physicians with knowledge and expertise in this area, including toxicologists, neurologists, rheumatologists and holistic doctors specializing in detoxification. This greatly aided in my search for methods that would work to remove the chemicals, as well as the silicone, from the body. In my quest for a cure, I had my own body on which to experiment.

At first I used supplements and fasting for detoxification and found that supplements that assisted in the removal of chemicals from the body helped. Immune boosting supplements were also very important in my recovery, as it was difficult to maintain my 100-hour-plus-work-week as a surgeon while chronically ill from viral or yeast infections. Several interviews I conducted on my radio show during this time significantly helped me to develop the *Silicone Immune Protocol*.[37] These included the interview with Dr. Andrew Campbell, one of the editors of *The International Journal of Occupational Medicine and Toxicology*'s special issue

---

[37] Kolb, Susan E. "Doctor, Are You Listening?" 1996. *Millennium Healthcare*. 19 Jan. 2009.
http://plastikos.com/documents/DoctorAreYouListeningTheSiliconeCatastrophe.pdf

covering the toxicology of silicone.[38]

My interview with Dr. Campbell helped me understand the toxicology of the silicone and chemicals in the silicone. The extensive effect that silicone and the chemicals contained in it can have on the neurological, immune and endocrine systems of the body was becoming increasingly clear to me. I then interviewed Dr. Lee Cowden,[39] an alternative medical doctor with experience in silicone detoxification methods to help me further understand the role of detoxification in this illness.

I also spoke with Dr. Arthur Brawer, a rheumatologist who saw the wisdom in holistic methods,[40] and Dr. David Perlmutter,[41] a holistic neurologist who was very familiar with silicone toxicity and neurological disease from implant exposure. I had the opportunity to interview many experts in detoxification including Dr. Michael Murray,[42] a prominent naturopath and expert in detoxification, who

[38] Brautbar, Nachman, Andrew Campbell and Aristo Vojdani, eds. *International Journal of Occupational Medicine and Toxicology*. Special Issue on Silicone Toxicity. 4 (1995).
[39] Cowden, W. Lee, Russ DiCarlo, and Burton Goldberg. *Longevity : An Alternative Medicine Definitive Guide*. New York: AlternativeMedicine.com Books, 2004.
[40] Brawer, Arthur E. *Holistic Harmony*. NJ: Vista, 1999.
[41] Perlmutter, David, and Carol Colman. *The Better Brain Book : The Best Tools for Improving Memory and Sharpness and for Preventing Aging of the Brain*. New York: Riverhead Books (Hardcover), 2004.
[42] Murray, Michael T., and Joseph E. Pizzorno. *Encyclopedia of Natural Medicine: Your Comprehensive, User-Friendly A-to-Z Guide to Treating More Than 70 Medical Conditions--from Arthritis to Varicose Veins, from Cancer to Heart Disease*. New York: Three Rivers P, 1997.

commented on the air that I had the only detoxification program for silicone toxicity that he had ever seen.

In 2007 and again in 2008, I interviewed Dr. Hildegarde Staninger, a toxicologist familiar with silicone who discovered silicone and high-density polyethylene in her investigation of Morgellons disease. Dr. Staninger's work raises the possibility that silicone could be associated with potentially life-threatening diseases.[43,44]

Attention to the immune system would become an important aspect of patient care and would be critical to my success in treating silicone-induced disease. The majority of my patients had immune system deficits especially involving natural killer T cells, which are important in immunity against fungi, viruses, and cancer. The majority of my patients also had evidence of systemic or local problems with candidiasis and mold. Later I was to find out the importance of biotoxins produced by the mold in their illness.

A fair percentage of the patients also had bacterial infections in the chest wall, which required treatment with antibiotics to alleviate. Unfortunately, if antibiotics were given without antifungal treatment, the symptoms related to biotoxins became more severe. Later studies would reveal

---

[43] Staninger, Hildegarde. *The Comprehensive Handbook of Hazardous Material: Regulations, Monitoring, Handling & Safety.* CRC Press. 2000.
[44] Staninger, Hildegarde. "Far-Infrared Radiant Heat (FIR RH) Type Remediation for Mold and Other Unique Diseases." Proc. of National Registry of Environmental Professionals Annual Conference, Nashville, TN. 2006.

that these patients have increased risk for many cancers including brain, lung, and colon cancer, but oddly enough, they had a reduced risk of breast cancer.[45,46]

My theory as to this reduced risk of breast cancer has to do with the triad of 1) pressure from the implant, 2) increased cytokine release within the chest wall, which includes cytokines such as tumor necrosis factor, and 3) increased silica within the chest wall which also may reduce the risk of cancer locally. I believe the increased risk of other cancers has to do with the immune deficit seen in these patients. Supplements that would help to increase natural killer T cells such as Transfer Factor Plus™ and EpiCor™ became very important in the protocol in order to reduce postoperative infectious complications.

The *Silicone Immune Protocol*[47] is posted on the Plastikos website (http://www.plastikos.com) and is updated frequently as more information becomes available regarding detoxification in the holistic and functional medicine literature. This is not a cookbook approach as each

---

[45] Zuckerman, Diana and Rachael Flynn. "Government Studies Link Breast Implants to Cancer, Lung Disease, and Suicide." *Breast Implant Info*. 2001. 19 Jan. 2009.
http://www.breastimplantinfo.org/what_know/implantgovstdy.html
[46] Briton, L. A., J. H. Lubin, M. C. Burdich, T. Colton, S. L. Brown, and R. N. Hoover. "Cancer Risk at Sites Other Than the Breast Following Augmentation Mammoplasty." *Annals of Epidemiology* 11 (2001): 248-56.
[47] Kolb, Susan E. "The Silicone Immune Protocol" 2007. *Millennium Healthcare*. 19 Jan. 2009.
http://www.plastikos.com/documents/SiliconeImmuneProtocol.pdf

patient has individual considerations that influence which portions of this protocol will be recommended.

For example, the doctor must determine which type of toxicity exists in the patient. For instance, the patient might be presenting symptoms from silicone toxicity, chemical toxicity, bio-toxicity, contributions from preexisting heavy metal and chemical toxicity not related to the implants or a combination of toxic conditions from more than one source. Diagnosis of the predominant toxicity is necessary in order to make recommendations that will help the patient remove the substances causing her symptoms.

If an incorrect diagnosis is made, the detoxification protocol is not likely to be successful and, in some cases, can be detrimental. The correct diagnosis is made with a careful history and physical exam, laboratory testing, hair analysis for toxic elements in some cases, and additional testing such as a visual contrast sensitivity exam to detect the presence of bio-toxins when indicated. *The Silicone Immune Protocol* addresses diet, exercise, nutrients, inflammation, immune function, detoxification, pain, infection, nerve pain, fatigue, insomnia and miscellaneous conditions.

Additional detoxification programs were developed to address patients who have problems with platinum, a metal used as a catalyst in older implants before research indicated it was toxic even in small amounts within the human body. Patients with platinum toxicity can be diagnosed both clinically and with the use of heavy metal and toxic hair analysis. In my clinical experience, patients with platinum toxicity may have adult onset asthma, neurological problems (to a greater degree than expected from silicone alone) and frequent multiple lipomas or fatty tumors.

Additional treatment information is available in the article "Transfer Factors in Clinical Medicine."[48] Transfer factors help transfer the ability to recognize a pathogen (i.e. bacteria or virus) in T cells that have not been in contact with the pathogen. I also refer many of my patients to an article written by Dr. Douglas Shanklin entitled "Inositol."[49] Dr. Shanklin discovered that the B vitamin, inositol, is a useful supplement in promoting the excretion of silicone from the body by converting it to silicate, which passes into the urine.

At a conference in Atlanta in 1997, on medical issues related to silicone breast implants, I had an opportunity to speak with a rheumatologist who had studied 3,000 women who had problems from their silicone breast implants from either leaking or rupturing. He had found 3,000 women who were positive for candidiasis or yeast after antibody testing. This was consistent with the theory that these women had an immune system deficient in T cell function.

Because the majority of my patients complained of fatigue, muscle aches, and mental clouding, which were

---

[48] Kolb, Susan E. "Transfer Factors in Clinical Medicine." 2008. *Millennium Healthcare*. 19 Jan. 2009.
http://www.plastikos.com/documents/TransferFactorsinClinicalMedicine.pdf
[49] Shanklin, Douglas. "Inositol." 23 Feb. 2008. *Millennium Healthcare*. 19 Jan. 2009 http://plastikos.com/documents/Inositol.pdf

common symptoms in a condition called fibromyalgia, I was treating this triad of symptoms with systemic anti-fungal agents if the patient had normal liver function tests. If the patient had abnormal liver function tests (which was fairly frequent as many of these patients overuse Tylenol™), I would use supplements such as Super Thistle X™ to normalize the liver function tests. Overgrowth of yeast or candidiasis was frequently seen in the intestine, throat, vagina and skin of these patients.

Many of these conditions, as well as some skin rashes, cleared up on the antifungal therapy. The use of the anti-fungal agents, either systemic or localized to the G.I. tract, around the time of surgery, was a very important adjunct to surgery. Patients who received antibiotics around the time of surgery without anti-fungal treatment would experience an exacerbation of the fatigue, muscle aches and mental clouding along with other symptoms such as G.I. bloating, vaginal yeast infections and shortness of breath. It was always a mystery to me why some surgeons who frequently performed explantation surgery did not make this connection and include anti-fungal therapy in their perioperative program.

Additional non-medication based anti-fungal therapies are listed in the *Silicone Immune Protocol* and are very useful in limiting yeast overgrowth in the intestine after the systemic anti-fungal drugs were discontinued. The role of diet in the prevention of yeast overgrowth is very important. Patients soon discover that a diet high in sugar or carbohydrates that are converted quickly to sugar result in recurrent symptoms of yeast overgrowth in the intestines, such as bloating and diarrhea.

I always emphasize the importance of using probiotics to replace the friendly gut bacteria that suppress yeast overgrowth, especially around the time of surgery or when on antibiotics. Whenever patients forget this important point, the yeast symptoms frequently recur, especially if they are not on the immune supplements designed to increase natural killer T cell function, such as Transfer Factor Plus™ and EpiCor™.

Immune system deficits require that patients follow a very healthy diet and lifestyle. The protocol for healing demands that they take every measure possible to assist their bodies in eliminating toxins.

SYMPTOMS OF SILICONE IMMUNE DISEASE

Endocrine System

Thyroid:
- Hair loss
- Constipation
- Weight Gain
- Dry Skin
- Low basal metabolic temperature

ADH:
- Dry Mouth
- Excessive thirst
- Shocks from static electricity
- Frequent urination

Adrenal:
- Low blood pressure
- Dizziness
- Passing out, especially when standing up quickly (orthostatic hypotension)
- Feeling as if you are dying

Sex Hormones:
- Irregular or lack of menses
- PMS
- Low sex drive

Neurological System

- Arrhythmias
- Cognitive Dysfunction
- Memory Loss
- Difficulty with Concentration
- Brain Fog
- Abnormal Brain MRI or Spectra Scan of the Brain
- Blurred Vision
- Sensory Loss
- Tingling
- Burning pain of extremities
- Muscle Weakness
- Balance Disturbance
- Burning Pain of the Chest Wall, Breast or Axilla
- Headaches
- Tremors
- Seizures

Immune System

Viral Infections:
- Mouth ulcers
- Herpes Simplex

Fungal Infections:
- Chronic Urinary Tract Infections
- Mouth Ulcers
- Shortness of Breath
- Depression
- Fungal Rashes

Bacterial Infections:
- Chronic Urinary Tract Infections
- Low grade fever
- Night Sweats
- Bronchitis
- Sinusitis
- Colitis
- Peridontal Disease

Autoimmune Disease (Intra-cellular bacteria)
- Rashes
- Joint Aches & Swelling
- Raynaud's Disease
- Dry eyes
- Dry mouth
- Photosensitivity
- Difficulty Swallowing
- Abnormal Blood Clotting

Other Symptoms:

- Restrictive Lung Disease
- Pericarditis
- Muscle Aches
- Chronic Fatigue
- Lymph Node Enlargement
- Mal-absorption Syndrome
- Food Allergies
- Multiple Lipomas (Platinum Exposure)
- New Onset Asthma (Platinum Exposure)

Beverly's Story

The Internet is truly a wondrous invention. While working as a missionary in Korea, Beverly found my website and contacted me. Her story not only shows how the world is becoming smaller every day, but also that with the correct spiritual guidance, you can be led anywhere in the world for help.

I have had patients who travel great distances, coming from every continent in the world, often finding me as a result of prayer. More often than not, when we meet for the first time in Atlanta, we immediately feel a kinship, as if we are already members of the same spiritual family. It was truly a pleasure taking care of Beverly and receiving advice from her worldly-wise new husband on how to dodge bullets, which may come my way.

> "I have been unable to keep a journal for some thirty years and have resisted reliving much of my adult life with good reason. One seldom desires to memorialize painful experiences. However, I will attempt to put together a

series of events that have led me to where I am today.

"My story begins fifty-three years ago when I was born into what I consider the perfect family situation with loving, supportive parents and two brothers. Ours was a good Christian home and we were taught to pray, read the Bible and live the Ten Commandments. Dad worked hard to provide for the needs of the family and Mom made living within our means an art form. She cooked, baked, sewed, knitted, grew a garden and pinched a penny better than anyone else I have ever known. Bargain hunting was one of our favorite adventures. Though our means were limited, we never knew what it was to want because we were taught to appreciate everything we had.

"We lived near the seashore (and we didn't have air conditioning), so we would spend every summer day at the beach, leaving the house just after our morning chores were completed and returning just in time to get dinner on the table for Dad's arrival home from work. The springs and falls were spent in the woods behind our house, exploring miles and miles of densely forested area, turning over every little rock, catching tadpoles to bring home and watch them grow, then releasing them when they had become 'croakers.' Fireflies were common houseguests as were many other 'critters' we would find and bring home. We always learned about them, and then put them back 'in the wild' because we felt it was wrong to destroy anything just because we were curious. We took our stewardship to care for the creations of the Lord very seriously.

"When I was five years old I began ballet lessons, which was quite a sacrifice for my parents. At the time I didn't notice that Mom's wardrobe was so conservative, or that we ate creative leftovers more often. What I remember is Mom going to lessons with me and sitting in the waiting room working on her knitting or reading a book, which she loved to do. And ballet . . . how I loved to dance. (I still dream of dancing today!) Life was gentle, kind and good. We had our challenges, but we were taught nothing was impossible with God.

"When I was sixteen years old, we left our home at the seashore and moved 2,000 miles to the West, leaving behind lifelong friends and extended family. I thought my heart would break, but we made new friends and talked to our family often. I discovered the advantages of attending a smaller school and living in a safer community, and soon things were even better than before. I had been very shy and the move to the new community gave me opportunities to blossom and open up in new ways.

"I had always felt like an ugly duckling since I was taller than everyone in my class . . . including the boys, and was very athletic and strong. In the new school I made friends easily and was given the nickname 'Barbie' after the Barbie™ doll because of my well proportioned figure. At one Drill Team performance, a less than polite man was heard to say, 'She's built like a brick shit house!' while goggling and pointing at me. When my friends told about the scene he had created, they also had to explain to me what he meant since I was unfamiliar with the term. I had a large chest and small waist, and the drill team costume showed it off. I always dressed to minimize my chest so I wouldn't be embarrassed by the stares and comments. I wore a 36D bra then.

"After graduating from high school, I attended college and met my first husband. He was a dashingly handsome 'older' student who had served in the Army and traveled the world. I thought he was very mature and well anchored. After a short courtship period he proposed and we married. Soon after the marriage I conceived and we had our first child. She was absolutely perfect...a 10 on the APGAR score and I couldn't have been happier. I had always dreamed of becoming a mother and raising my own children. My childhood experience had been so perfect, and I wanted to give my baby the same love and support I had been given by my parents.

"My loving husband soon showed his true colors. We had attended birthing classes together and decided I would nurse our baby for health benefits as well as cost savings. As a side benefit to him, my already large breasts became huge with the milk. I remember when my daughter was 2 months old he decided she didn't need to be fed during the night anymore. When my precious baby cried, I was forced to lie in my bed and listen until she finally would stop. I remember crying along with her, then lying awake hoping to hear a breath or a whimper to know she was still alive. Daytime feedings became unbearable as he would stand next to me and make remarks about how the baby was getting in his way or that he resented sharing 'his' breasts with the baby.

"Because he had isolated me from my family and friends I had nowhere to go and no one to talk to. I had always been a very prayerful person, so I turned to God for help and protection. After six months of nursing I finally gave up and switched to formula, and my breasts returned to normal. They were a little saggier than pre-pregnancy and still substantial (34D), but my husband wasn't satisfied. He would always talk about women with big breasts and say how much he missed mine.

"Three and one half years later I conceived and gave birth to another perfect baby girl. My breasts again became huge and I had enough milk for the neighborhood! Luckily he had matured some and was working full time so I had a little better experience with nursing and taking care of this baby. I nursed her for nine months before he convinced me it was time to stop. When my milk dried up, my breasts were still very substantial, just two babies softer. I was still a 34C/D at the time and quite thin, so I was very well proportioned.

"My loving husband started telling me about all the beautiful big-breasted women he would meet as a police officer (one happened to be a high school friend of mine) and lamented about how much he missed my big breasts. I remember one day in particular when he called on the phone and asked us to meet him for lunch at his 'favorite lunch restaurant.' I dressed our two girls up for Daddy and we drove to meet him for lunch. When we arrived he was inside with one of his friends, a fellow police officer, and they were flirting with the waitresses at their table, which was very commonplace. As we were eating lunch, he announced why we had been invited to that restaurant . . . he wanted me to see the waitress with the lovely breasts. Numerous other 'sightings' and photos of women with big breasts were to follow this event.

"At the time of our marriage in 1976, we had chosen to visit with a family practice doctor, who was the father of a college friend. This doctor seemed to be very personable and knowledgeable and was willing to work with my desire to go 'natural' with health care choices. We had been involved in a car accident in 1977 when our first baby was six months old, and I had sustained some serious injuries which left me unable to have any more children, or so said the three different OB/GYN doctors I had seen. The family doctor worked with me while I mixed herbs and made potions to drink that would curl a frog's toes! But after three years I was able to conceive our second child.

"My husband became aware that our doctor had performed breast augmentation on both of his daughters and was doing the surgery in his clinic. He presented me with the idea of having the same surgery because, 'It must be safe. He has done the surgery on his own daughters.' For years I had been eating a very healthy diet, mostly organic foods with whole grains and vegetables. I used herbs to address any health concerns and all natural home and health care products. The last thing I wanted to do was consider putting silicone in my body, but his pressure was consistent and constant.

"I still remember how excited he and the doctor were at the consultation appointment. I felt as though I was at a funeral and they were at a party. I was persuaded this 'small sacrifice' would save my marriage, so I consented to undergo surgery in 1980. My husband had already been involved in at least two extramarital affairs at that point, and he had convinced me it was my fault he had wandered. I remember how excited he was for the surgery. He usually complained about every penny spent but he had scraped together a loan for the $800 surgery, and it was 'a great investment' for him.

"My surgery was performed in the doctor's office one evening after office hours. The silicone implants were placed under the breast tissue, above the muscle through incisions made under the breast. I recovered in record time with no complications. Other than my husband and the doctor, no one knew I had the surgery. I was too ashamed to tell anyone and I really didn't look much different from before surgery. My own mother did not notice any difference, but my husband was happy. At least for a little while, until he returned to his wandering ways.

"I continued to eat a very healthy diet and maintained a high level of activity. My diet included an array of natural vitamins and supplements with high doses of vitamin E to encourage elasticity and prevent scarring. Within two years my breasts were 'encapsulating' and the doctor 'popped' the capsules manually several times in the doctor's office. Other than not having a menstrual period (which had been caused by the auto accident in 1977) my health was very good. I had a few small annoyances like eczema, frequent sore throats that resulted in the removal of my tonsils at age twenty-eight and a constant lump in my throat, for which there was no explanation. But generally I felt well and had energy to spare.

"In 1983 I gave birth to a beautiful boy. The birth was more difficult than the first two as he was a double footling breech (I had him vaginally), and I hemorrhaged with the delivery of the placenta. He was very healthy, though a little smaller than my first two babies, and he jaundiced the week after birth. He also had clubfeet that were treated with casts and special shoes with a brace. He did well on my milk for five months but then began to have digestive problems, so he was switched to certified goats milk (purchased at a local goat dairy) at six months.

"He was healthy in every other way and did well as he was introduced to whole foods. Keep in mind; I fed my babies only whole, pure foods, organic if possible. I cleaned the food, cooked it and ground it for the children myself, mixed with herbs and supplements to give them the greatest nutrition possible. So they had custom diets based on their individual needs and conditions.

"After the birth of my son I developed several lumps in my right breast that my doctor was 'watching.' Through my years of natural health care I had great success with using clay, so I packed the breast faithfully day and night over a period of several months and the lumps disappeared. Both breasts were encapsulated and hard after breastfeeding but I couldn't bear the thought of having them 'popped' again, and we had moved to an area 200 miles away from the implanting doctor.

"In 1985 our last child was born. She was also a double footling breech so she was born cesarean section under great protest from me. The hospital would not allow her to be delivered 'naturally.' She was my second biggest baby and very healthy at birth. She also was jaundiced in her first week and had the clubfeet, but she nursed very well and thrived on my milk for eight months. She did not display the stomach disturbances that my son had, though she constantly had swollen lymph nodes.

"When I stopped nursing, I had developed several lumps in each breast, which were hard and sensitive. I treated them with the clay as I had done before, but they did not go away this time. And for some strange reason, I had started reacting to the clay. Wherever I placed the clay on my body, my skin would burn within minutes of applying it. I surmised I had developed sensitivity to the clay. I had also become more sensitive to all chemicals and even medicines over the past five years, though I continued to eat healthy foods and eliminated all possible toxins and chemicals from my environment.

"My breasts were completely encapsulated at that point, which made the lumps even more prominent and uncomfortable. I visited several doctors through the HMO we were using for health care. They wanted to remove and biopsy the lumps but would not address the implant issue. I was afraid of what might be under the implants and a possible rupture during surgery but the doctors would not even discuss those concerns with me.

"In 1990, I decided it was time to take action. I knew my insurance wouldn't touch my problem, but I needed to resolve the issue. Earlier that year I had lost a maternal aunt to breast cancer, and I was worried about my health. My mother had dealt with breast lumps all of her adult life, and I had begun the lumps at the tender age of eighteen, with my first lumpectomy the summer I graduated from high school.

"All things considered, I wanted those implants and the lumps removed all together, not one without the other. I decided I wanted to have the implants and all the breast tissue removed so I wouldn't have any danger of cancer, and have reconstructive implants placed in at the same time. You know, the 'safe' kind (saline) that lasted a lifetime.

"The doctor I found to do the surgery was a plastic surgeon 'friend' who had been my ecclesiastical leader in my college days. He was pleased to see me and told me of the latest reconstructive implants that were safe and would last forever. I remember him telling me what a 'sexy senior citizen' I would be with these implants (a shock from a spiritual leader under any circumstances) and virtually 100% guarantee of never developing breast cancer, since he would place the implants under the muscle. No need for mammograms either. I was sold.

"The implants he recommended were double lumen with saline in the outside lumen and a small amount of silicone injected into a lumen in the middle of the saline to 'even things out' after removing the breast and old scar tissues. I questioned the valve system that was used to fill the inside lumen, and he said it was perfectly safe and 'self sealing.' No chance of leakage. He was the expert, I didn't know anything about implants, and he was a friend who had been a spiritual leader. What was there not to trust?

"The lumps were to be evaluated at the lab. He was supposed to check the old implants for leaks, and everything was to be cleaned out, so I was pleased. The doctor and my husband worked out the details on financing this adventure ($2,600.00 this go) and my husband requested the 'Dolly Parton' size, which I put a stop to. I didn't want to be any larger, just problem free. Even at that, the implants were a special order because they were so new and so large. Surgery was scheduled and my husband took out another loan to cover the cost. He balked at buying school clothing for the children, but he was eager to finance 'his' new breasts!

"The surgery was performed in the doctor's 'surgery suite' at his office. I again did very well and went back to work three days after surgery with little to no pain. At the first follow-up visit I asked about the lab work on the lumps to which he replied they were fine, and he didn't need to send them to the lab. Just plugged milk glands. I then asked about the old implants, and he said they were in 'good shape' just encapsulated.

"Then I asked about the removal of the tissue to which he replied that he had left a 'very thin layer' under the nipples for smoothness and if there were ever a problem with lumps then it would be very localized and easy to take care of. Any cancer threat was 'gone.' I had just bought a lifetime of carefree breast cancer prevention. What a deal!

"In 1986, I had undergone a vaginal hysterectomy but didn't think anything of it since my uterus had been damaged in the car accident in 1977, and I had never had a menstrual period after that time. Then there were all the irregularities with the endocrine system and constant vaginal yeast infections, which I blamed on the damage to the uterus.

"I also had developed 'knots' in my neck and back, which I blamed on the old whiplash from a car accident way back. I blamed my anxiety and inability to sleep on my husband's incessant flirting and affairs with other women and his abusive treatment of the children and me. I had an explanation for everything.

"In 1995, I went to the doctor because the lump in my throat was so bad I felt like I was gagging all the time, and I was so tired I couldn't function. I thought it might be my thyroid. I was an area manager for a large retail chain working 60 to 70 hours per week, serving as a local elected official, mothering four children and trying to cope with a less than ideal marriage. I was shocked when the doctor found an ovarian cyst and scheduled me for surgery immediately. When my uterus had been removed in 1986, the ovaries had been left 'just in case they decided to work' and I refused hormone replacement therapy. I had developed a thirteen-pound tumor on the right ovary.

"Following that surgery my health continued to decline, as did my marriage. Over the next few years I dealt with some strange things like Bell's palsy, increasing muscle 'cramps' and tightness, numbness in my limbs, digestive disturbances, night sweats, headaches and a host of other strange symptoms. Instead of doing aerobics and lifting weights as I had enjoyed in the past, I struggled just to walk around the neighborhood.

"I had changed my profession from retail management to real estate in an attempt to find more flexibility to cover all of my responsibilities. I was in pain all the time but was afraid to take anything for it because I reacted negatively to everything I tried. One morning in 2000, I ended up at the hospital emergency room with chest and arm pain and numbness. I was afraid I might be having a heart attack, but thankfully it wasn't my heart. I was referred to an internal medicine specialist, and he formally diagnosed me with fibromyalgia.

"Things continued to go downhill until I hit 'rock bottom' in 2001. My husband, after seven affairs that I knew of, announced he was leaving me for another woman, but not before we had refinanced our home to include all of 'our' consolidated debts in the mortgage. What a wonderful guy...he left me the house...and the payment too! No alimony, or financial help. My fibromyalgia was so bad at that time that I was unable to work, and the stress of providing for my children and myself put me flat on my back in bed. In real estate if you don't work, you don't earn any money! From head to toe, I was a complete mess.

"The Lord had been my constant help and companion, and once again, though more literally then ever before, I turned to him for help. I had a family to care for, no health insurance, no income and no one to do it for me. Through daily miracles he got me out of bed and back on my feet enough to find a way to move on. Some 'old deals' closed, and I had a little money to work with until I was able to get back on my feet a bit. My children were wonderful, and I was reunited with my family after being kept away from them for twenty-five years. Things were looking up. I even began dating a bit.

"With no health insurance, I relied on the help of a nutritionist and a massage therapist, both women whom I had become friends with through the years. They got me going and again I enjoyed success in earning a living. My relationship with my children was better than ever, and I was enjoying life again. The fibromyalgia, however, constantly reminded me that I was limited in what I could do. Though my spirit wanted to fly, my body kept me cautiously grounded.

"In 2003, at the age of forty-nine, I met my second husband . . . on the Internet. He is truly a Godsend, a literal gift from God. He had lost his dear wife of forty years to cancer and was 'testing the waters' to see if he might find a companion to share adventures with for the rest of his life. Though he is seventeen years my senior he is vital and 'young at heart.' We made a wonderful connection and he asked me to be his wife, knowing up front I struggled with health issues. On our honeymoon we played a game called 'Scars and Missing Parts.' Use your imagination. Anyway, he won the scars and I won the missing parts. (I counted each breast separately!)

"Right after the honeymoon we began searching for a doctor to help with the fibromyalgia, and I interviewed several who were supposed to be 'specialists.' Our search led us to an M.D./N.D. 150 miles from our home. We made an appointment to meet with her and she spent an hour with us, answering all of our questions and evaluating all of my hundreds of symptoms. She ordered lab tests and recommended vitamins, supplements and treatments based on her exam and the results of the lab tests.

"I have always been sensitive to cold weather, but after our marriage I moved to my husband's home at an altitude of 7000 feet above sea level where the weather hits extremes in heat and cold. My first winter was spent mostly in bed and in pain. Great way to start a marriage! But my husband had committed to dedicate his time and means to helping me get well and that he did. Under the care of my new doctor, I began to improve gradually but steadily.

"At one point we were driving the 300-miles round trip two times per week for treatments, but the commitment paid off. Eventually, I was able to go one day without having to go back to bed, then two. After two and a half years of treatment, I was well enough to begin some adventures. We had to adhere to great preventative measures and caution with foods and the environment, but we had learned my 'limits' to a great degree.

"One of our great adventures led us to accept a call to serve a volunteer church mission overseas in Korea. We visited with our doctors who noted any applicable limitations and recommendations for our service. As part of the process I was asked to have a mammogram, so I returned to the implanting surgeon for a check up. He said everything was fine and no mammogram was needed since all the breast tissue had been removed. I asked about the burning pain and popping in my breasts, and he said it must be the fibromyalgia. He should know.

"So we packed our two suitcases each (mine filled with vitamin supplements, natural health and personal care items that would be unavailable there, plus my portable treatment machine) and boarded an airplane. We planned our activities around my limitations and informed our leaders of my need for flexibility. Despite fatigue and days when I couldn't do anything, things went well for seven months until I developed white spots under every fingernail, which I had never had before; nor had I sustained any injury. Until then, I had blamed every unusual symptom on the fibromyalgia, but I couldn't find any reference or connection between fibro and white spots. I increased my research and found information that mentioned silicone poisoning as a possible cause.

"I was horrified and a little confused. My implants were silicone, or so I had been told. I contacted the implanting surgeon and asked what I should do. He said, 'Do nothing. Your implants are silicone and if they rupture the saline will be contained in the pocket until it is absorbed into the body.' By that time I had read enough to know that saline wasn't the innocent substance it had been presented to be and that a rupture could be devastating. I requested a copy of my operative records and after much resistance, they agreed to send my records via mail.

"The following week I was showering and massaging my breast and I felt a pop, sort of like popping a bubble gum bubble in your mouth. I knew I was in big trouble. I hadn't told my husband what I had discovered yet because I wasn't certain I was correct. Fear took over and I told him we needed to talk about what was going on. This sweet man had been through so much with me over the previous three years, and now I had to tell him I thought I had another problem. After we talked, he began his own Internet research, and we both were horrified to find that the symptoms I had been dealing with over the past many years were likely aggravated, if not entirely caused, by the implants.

"When my medical records arrived from the implanting surgeon, I was further horrified. The records showed the implants were double lumen, but with silicone in the outside lumen and saline in the inner lumen. Further, his operative notes did not mention removing any breast or scar tissue, just removing the old implants and putting the new ones in under the muscle. At that point, I had no idea what I was dealing with. He had told me that my breast tissue was gone and that I had saline filled implants with a small amount of silicone in the center that couldn't possibly leak, which he had reiterated in multiple follow-up visits over the years. But the records told another story.

"After years of suffering from seemingly endless, unrelated problems, I finally felt I had found the culprit to my declining health. My husband and I agreed that I could not wait until our mission was completed to address this problem, so we began searching for a doctor to remove the implants properly. I had learned they needed to be removed 'en bloc' along with any trace of scar tissue or damage and, heaven forbid, leaking silicone.

"Finding a physician in Korea was next to impossible since we do not speak the language, and the English-speaking health clinic had no idea what I was talking about when I called to inquire about their services. We determined we would need to return to the USA for surgery as soon as possible. Coincidentally, my son was being married in mid-May, and we had planned an approved trip home for the wedding. We decided to return four weeks early for surgery.

"As I set about selecting a doctor, I put up my petition to God to guide and direct me to the best physician for my needs. Because of my connection to alternative medicine and natural health care, I had been favorably impressed by Dr. Susan Kolb's detailed explanation of the problem and her approach, not only to proper removal of the implants, but the whole-body approach to detoxification and healing.

"Early in my research, I felt drawn to her approach and methods of healing, but wanting to be certain she was the right choice for me, I wrote to several doctors and evaluated their responses. It did not come as a surprise when Dr. Kolb's response was the most appropriate. I moved forward with plans to schedule surgery and finalize travel.

"Throughout my life I have been aware of the hand of God leading me and confirming when I have made a correct choice. This was especially evident as we prepared to make the trip to the USA and have the surgery done. One question we had was where we would stay for the ten days to two weeks we needed to be in Atlanta. By no coincidence, we heard from some friends who live in Chicago and owned a second home in

Newnan, GA. When they heard about my surgery, they not only offered to have us stay with them, but insisted they would be gravely offended if we didn't.

"We flew into the Atlanta airport on a Tuesday and visited with Dr. Kolb the next day for the consultation. When we met I felt like I had known her for a very long time. She patiently answered all of my many questions, and we spoke candidly about my expectations, future options and the outcome of the surgery. I knew I had been led to her to partner in my healing, and I knew I would be able to recover in time.

"Because my surgery was being covered by insurance (another miracle), it was to be done in the hospital. On Thursday we registered at the hospital and had a breast ultrasound done. The ultrasound showed both implants were ruptured, and the right capsule also. On Friday we met for the pre-op appointment, and Dr. Kolb again spent a great deal of time with us, answering all of our questions and calming all of my fears. I asked her to check a 'funny' spot on my right cheek, which we determined she would remove during surgery and have the lab analyze along with the implants and capsules. She expected surgery to last for around five to six hours.

"Mine was the first surgery scheduled on Monday morning, so we left the house in Newnan around 4:30 AM to get to the hospital on time. Dr. Kolb came in to visit with my husband and me one last time before surgery, and I was off to sleepy land. Our friends came to the hospital to wait with my husband during surgery, which was a good thing, because the surgery ended up lasting ten hours. Dr. Kolb found the grossly ruptured implant and capsule in the right breast as expected and spent hours removing silicone that had migrated throughout my chest. She also repaired the damaged chest wall muscles.

"When she got into the left side, she found the original capsule had not been removed and was filled with fluid...something the ultrasound technician had missed completely. The chest muscles were badly damaged and there was evidence of old silicone damage. She also removed the enlarged lymph nodes under both arms to prevent any future problems with built up silicone in the nodes. All tissue and the implants were sent to the lab for analysis.

"When I awakened, I was in an observation room with my husband by my side. We spent the night at the hospital where my vital signs were monitored, and I was released the next morning with drains in both breasts. I rested very comfortably at the home of our friends and did not need to take the pain medicine after the second day. I slept a lot, which was a blessing, since sleeplessness was one of the worst symptoms I had dealt with for years.

"The day after surgery the permanent knots in my shoulders (I had named them Fred and Fredonia) and neck were gone. Within a week my husband said he could see and feel a difference in my skin, and the anxiety that I had suffered for years was gone. The improvement in my health was noticeable to my husband as well as rapid. At long last I finally felt freed from the poison I knew was damaging my health.

"The drains were removed after seven days and I was amazed at how good my breasts looked. Dr. Kolb did a lift at the time of surgery to remove all the extra skin associated with housing those silicone wonders, and I went from a 36DD with implants to a 36 A/B after surgery.

My breasts feel and look great and they are no longer under my chin! They sit nicely on my chest where they should be.

"It has been four and a half months since surgery, and we are back in Korea, busier than ever. I am gaining health and strength every week. I still have my 'down' days, but they are less severe and less frequent than before. I still deal with some strange symptoms, but I know I need to be patient in my recovery. It took me twenty-seven years to get this sick and I guess I can't expect everything to disappear overnight...though I'd like it to!

"To summarize my experience, I made a very poor decision years ago that has plagued me for decades. No matter who influenced me or why I made the decision, it is mine. I own it. I am the only one who will have to answer to God for what I did to his gift to me...my body. I have paid the price for that decision for many years and, through the infinite love and the grace of God, I will partner with him, asking for forgiveness and pleading for the miracle of restored health. As one of my favorite songs says, 'For with God nothing is impossible.'

"I know God brought Dr. Kolb into my life as a gift to me and as a way to begin healing. I have been given a much better than average chance to begin the healing process through her God-given gift of healing. It is now up to me to seek out and incorporate the things that will bolster my health and continue to clean out my body."

-4-
SALINE IMPLANT DISEASE

"What you do not know will not hurt you, it will kill you."
Anonymous.
(Rumored to be on the wall behind the desk
of a prominent general.)

Saline Implant Disease is a different syndrome than Silicone Immune Disease, although some of the symptoms are similar. Both groups usually exhibit between twenty and thirty symptoms, often involving most of the body's physiological systems, especially the endocrine system, the immune system and the neurological system.

At first I suspected that the silicone shell of the saline implants was the primary culprit, but after reading a scientific article which reported that the amount of silicon in the scar capsules surrounding smooth silicone gel implants contained one hundred times more silicon than the capsules surrounding smooth saline implants, I began to question my theory[1]. From pathology reports, it also appeared that silicone from textured shells of saline implants may have flaked off and become embedded in the scar capsule. From there it could perhaps make its way into the lymphatic system and thereby interact with the immune system. Because most of saline breast implant illness patients did not have a primary autoimmune picture with rashes and joint aches as prominent symptoms, I could not see how silicone alone was the culprit.

I experienced a breakthrough discovery in my quest for answers when a computer technician from the United States Center for Disease Control, which is headquartered in Atlanta, became my patient. I found it ironic to see a patient from the CDC on my schedule whose chief complaint was an infection since I am a plastic surgeon. For years, the CDC clinic doctors had been sending me patients for wounds and hand injuries, and as my reputation developed for treating carpal tunnel syndrome without surgery, I began seeing more patients with that condition.

My CDC doctors are delightful patients in that they extensively research their medical conditions and share their findings with me. They are a highly intelligent group of individuals, more than willing to explore alternative treatments, and they often achieve outstanding results. So

---

[1] Schnur, Paul L. "Silicon Analysis of Breast and Periprosthetic Capsular Tissue from Patients with Saline or Silicone Gel Breast Implants." *Plastic and Reconstructive Surgery Journal* 98 (1996): 798-803.

when a computer technician who had become extremely ill with sick building syndrome sought my help, I was not surprised when she began to educate me regarding this newly emerging disease. She introduced me to the concept of biotoxins produced by mold in the environment, which in certain genetically predisposed individuals can cause major disruption of the endocrine, immune and neurological systems.

I researched the literature on biotoxins, including the work of Dr. Ritchie Shoemaker, the author of a book called *Mold Warriors*,[2] and had the opportunity to interview Dr. Shoemaker on my radio show.[3] During the interview, I mentioned to Dr. Shoemaker that some of my patients had mold growing in or around their breast implants. He commented that he had never heard of mold growing inside the chest wall and said, "I bet those patients are really ill." I replied that they frequently came to the clinic in wheelchairs.

After speaking with Dr. Shoemaker and reading his material, I was able to differentiate between the biotoxicity I was seeing in my saline implant patients from the chemical and silicone toxicity I was seeing in my silicone gel breast implant patients.

Around the same time, I received an urgent phone call

---

[2] Shoemaker, Ritchie C., James Schaller, and Patti Schmidt. *Mold Warriors: Fighting America's Hidden Health Threat.* Baltimore: Gateway P, 2005.
[3] "Shoemaker Interview," *Temple of Health Radio Program.* Telephone interview. 2005.

from a concerned father from Lake Charles, Louisiana, who told me his daughter was very ill and hardly able to get out of bed. She had developed severe joint pain, muscle pain, mental clouding, rashes and burning pain around her breast implants upon returning to a home full of mold contamination after the evacuation during Hurricane Rita.

None of the doctors in Lake Charles were able to help her. Fortunately, I was able to diagnose her illness and prescribe treatment that would help her. After removal of her breast implants and capsules, treatment for detoxification of the biotoxins and anti-fungal treatment for the mold growing within her chest wall, her health improved significantly.

Observations of similarly affected patients lead me to question what happens when a woman with saline implants is exposed to an environment rich in mold spores. The contaminants may reach the breast implants via the bloodstream after the spores are inhaled. I have encountered several patients, who after evacuating from hurricanes, returned to their homes to sleep on moldy mattresses and quickly developed a serious disease consistent with sick building syndrome, but with the sick building inside their chest wall. More study is needed to determine if these patients simply had mold around their implants or also had mold inside their implants.

The majority of my saline patients had isolated biotoxicity symptoms including reduced alpha MSH levels (due to the damaged leptin receptors in the hypothalamus) and abnormal visual contrast sensitivity tests (due to the neurotoxicity of the biotoxin affecting the optic nerve). I later understood that some of my silicone gel breast implant patients had combination of chemical toxicity and biotoxicity, and that was why there was a more varied clinical picture in these patients. I found the protocols for detoxification of biotoxins to be useful additions for the *Silicone Immune Protocol*.[4]

Of course, since these patients had the "sick building syndrome" inside their chest walls, if anti-fungal therapy was not used around the time of surgery, it took them a long time to get well. In the absence of anti-fungal treatment, the conditions of stress associated with surgery, as well as the use of antibiotics around the time of surgery, were very likely to cause accelerated growth of mold or fungus in the chest wall.

In certain susceptible individuals, who may have a genetic inability to rid the body of the biotoxins, it does not take much mold within the body to produce biotoxins to the degree that the patient becomes very ill. Indeed, if systemic anti-fungal therapy is not begun before surgery, surgery itself may lead to increased release of biotoxins that exacerbate the disease.

For patients with only one saline implant that is growing mold either in or around the implant, we see the neurological symptoms isolated to that side of the body. For

---

[4] Kolb, Susan E. "The Silicone Immune Protocol" 2007. *Millennium Healthcare*. 19 Jan. 2009.
http://www.plastikos.com/documents/SiliconeImmuneProtocol.pdf

patients with an infected left breast implant, we frequently see cardiac arrhythmias as the submuscular implant is very close to the heart. Manipulation of the implant and scar capsule during surgery increases these arrhythmias, whereas manipulation of the right-sided implant does not.

Patients with only one contaminated implant show abnormal visual contrast sensitivities on the same side as the affected implant. This would indicate that the biotoxins do not travel via the bloodstream under normal circumstances. The chemistry of the biotoxins is such that they are readily incorporated into cell walls, especially those involving nerves. This would explain heart arrhythmias when the left implant (which is over the heart) is affected, but not when the implant on the right side (which is not over the heart) is affected.

Unfortunately, we do not currently have a way to measure biotoxins either in the capsular tissue or in the blood. Instead, we measure the effect of biotoxins, which can lower the alpha MSH hormone and can also cause an abnormal visual contrast sensitivity test, as biotoxins are neurotoxins. Patients with this disease frequently complain of blurred vision that comes and goes.

Ophthalmologists are usually unable to ascertain the cause of the blurred vision with tests normally used. Surgeons who fail to use drains for a sufficient period of time or fail to remove the entire scar capsule which contains the mold contamination or do not treat the patient with anti-fungal agents may fail to resolve the patient's symptoms, and in some cases, exacerbate biotoxin related symptoms after surgery.

Bacterial infection generally presents with localized or radiating tenderness and burning pain while fungal infection can be more difficult to diagnose. In some cases, fungal infections produce minimal local discomfort, while in other cases, biotoxins released by the mold or fungus produce a burning pain that affects the local sensory nerves. Some cases of fungal contamination are diagnosed only by the systemic symptoms.

According to the medical literature on sick building syndrome, approximately one-fourth of the population is susceptible to illness caused by mold biotoxins.[5] This vulnerability is based on a genetic inability to detoxify the biotoxin. Therefore, when the implant becomes contaminated with fungus, either due to growth of the fungus in or around the implant after the surgery or after a valve defect, or in some cases, exposure to mold in the environment, the patient becomes ill with a systemic disease.

I have seen patients who became ill shortly after implantation surgery, most likely from mold spores contaminating the saline implant during surgery. This is less likely to happen if the surgeon uses a closed saline system during surgery, rather than drawing up saline from a bowl on the back table where mold spores can settle. It is also

---

[5] Shoemaker, Ritchie C. and King-Teh Lin. "The Ever-Expanding Data Base on Pathophysiology of Illness Caused by Exposure to Water-Damaged Buildings." Jan. 2008. *Indoor Environment Connection.* 24 Jan. 2009 http://www.schoolmoldhelp.org/images/stories/shoemaker-lin-Jan08.pdf p.4

advisable to use a no touch technique when handling the implant. I have even seen breast scar capsules with "rice granules," around them on one side only, likely some parasitic form due to contamination at surgery.

A more common situation is the development of fungal contamination inside the implant due to a valve defect often following trauma to the chest wall. Such trauma can occur as a result of a motor vehicle accident or even a mammogram and causes a minor deflation of the saline implant. Once the valve mechanism becomes incompetent, even for a brief time, it appears that the saline inside the implant becomes a medium for fungal growth. It is no surprise that moisture in the bag inside the chest wall is susceptible to fungal and bacterial contamination especially if the valve has been compromised.

Clinical diagnosis of fungal infections can be very difficult if one relies on microbiological cultures. Dr. Pierre Blais, a biochemist in Canada who specializes in the analysis of breast implants, has written extensively on this problem.[6] Bacterial cultures may very well be positive when capsular tissue is cultured if the patient has not been pretreated with antibiotics.

Because I currently treat many of these patients with antibiotics before surgery, these bacterial cultures now are usually negative. Fungal cultures are particularly difficult to

---

[6] Blais, Pierre. "Saline Filled Breast Implants: A Continuing Area of Concern." Mar. 2000. FDA Advisory Committee on Saline Filled Breast Implants. 24 Jan. 2009.
http://implants.clic.net/tony/blais/037.html

grow from capsular material, and though such cultures eventually do grow fungus, it is often read as an environmental contaminant and not as a pathogen. It may be, however, that the fungus growing out of the culture is responsible for making the patient ill.

The fungus is likely producing a biotoxin that the patient is unable to detoxify due to a genetic defect. It does not take much fungal growth to create a significant amount of biotoxin. The biotoxin is very lipophilic, or lipid loving, and incorporates easily into cell wall membranes throughout the body.

Medical mycologists have found mold inside the implants and suspect that mold is also in the scar capsule surrounding the implant. It may, however, require DNA typing of the capsular tissue to identify the mold in the capsule. I am currently working with medical mycologists to grow and identify fungal elements within the saline component of the implant.

According to Dr. Shoemaker, the biotoxin produces excessive cytokine levels, which damage leptin receptors in the hypothalamus and lower alpha MSH levels. The biotoxin disrupts the endocrine system via the hypothalamus, the immune system and the neurological system.[7]

---

[7] Schmidt, Patti. "New Theory Links Neurotoxins with Chronic Fatigue Syndrome, Lyme, MCS and Other Mystery Illnesses." *ProHealth Wellness Portal.* 29 Nov. 2002. 24 Jan. 2009
http://www.prohealth.com//library/showArticle.cfm?libid=8849

The endocrine system symptoms include frequent urination and thirst, secondary to an anti-diuretic hormone (ADH) deficiency as well as fatigue, easy weight gain, constipation, hair loss and dry skin secondary to a secondary thyroid deficiency. A low basal metabolic temperature taken in the morning before rising can easily diagnose a thyroid deficiency, but the diagnosis is considered subclinical because the thyroid function tests are not usually abnormal, although the free T4 is frequently in the low normal range.

Adrenal insufficiency is easily diagnosed with an abnormal pupillary response to light due to muscle fatigue of the pupillary sphincter. Adrenal symptoms often include dizziness especially when getting up quickly, weakness and a feeling that one is dying. Increasing intake of salt can be beneficial.

If sex hormones are also low, we see menstrual irregularities in some women and premature menopause in others. Reduced alpha MSH levels can also produce sleep disturbance because of lowered melatonin, chronic pain due to lowered endorphin production and malabsorption in intestine also known as "leaky gut" syndrome.[8]

High cytokine levels also can lead to restricted blood flow and lowered oxygen levels presenting as fatigue, muscle cramps and shortness of breath. And increased levels of

---

[8] Koontz, D., J. Hinze, et al. "Leaky Gut Syndrome, Origins, Effects and Therapies, The Medical Link Between Dysbiosis and many Major Ailments." *The Herbal Pharm* 19 (1999).

cytokines can produce systemic inflammation of the brain, nerves, muscle, lungs and joints.

Biotoxins are often neurotoxins and can be measured with a test called a visual contrast sensitivity test. In patients with a certain genetic susceptibility, additional neurological problems occur because some patients develop antibodies to myelin basic protein (which affects neurological function), gliadin (which affects digestion), cardiolipins (which affect blood clotting), and triggering of the complement immune pathway with elevated C3 A levels.

Biotoxins also affect the immune system. White blood cells lose regulation of cytokine response so that recovery from infectious diseases may be delayed. Detoxification of the mold biotoxins is accomplished primarily with the use of butyrate, an essential fatty acid which displaces the biotoxin from the cell membrane, and cholestyamine, a fiber which binds the biotoxin in the gut and aides removal from the body.

Other detoxification procedures such as IV glutathione, Reconastat™, Well BetX™, and ionic foot baths also can help to speed up the detoxification process. Systemic antifungal therapy is very important in the treatment of this disease. Without antifungal therapy, recovery is significantly slower, especially if antibiotics are given around the time of the explantation surgery.

Although silicone toxicity or siliconosis is found more frequently in patients with leaking silicone gel implants than in patients with saline implants, textured saline implants may present silicone to the immune system as particles break off from the implants, especially with rough handling from trauma, including mammograms. Patients with certain genetic HLA types such as HLA DR 53 may be more susceptible to autoimmune diseases from silicone exposure.[9] Therefore, patients with these HLA types might be advised to avoid silicone implants.

There is also evidence of a biofilm of protein material on the surface of the implant that may predispose the areas of the body that come into contact with it to develop bacterial and or fungal infections. When scar tissue invades the valve mechanism, these bacteria and other microorganisms can easily track into the saline implant. Studies reveal that the saline solution contained within the implants can support the growth of these microorganisms,[10] and indeed this is what we find when we look inside the saline implants removed from patients with clinical signs and symptoms of chest wall infection.

The biotoxins produced by mold contamination are also associated with severe depression and anxiety.[11] On more than one occasion a woman has called my office on the verge of suicide. Kathryn Gordon, whose story was featured in

---

[9] Young, V. L., J. R. Nemecek, B. D. Schwartz, D. L. Phelan, and M. W. Schorr. "HLA Typing in Women with and without Silicone Gel-filled Breast Implants." *Current Topics in Microbiology and Immunology* 210 (1996): 209-225.
[10] Young, V. Leroy, M. Cathreine Hertl, Patrick R. Murray, John Jensen, Holly Witt, Maria Schorr, and M. A. Watson. "Microbial Growth Inside Saline-Filled Breast Implants." *Plastic and Reconstructive Surgery Journal* 100 (1997): 182-96.
[11] Potera, Carol. "Mental Health: Molding a Link to Depression." *PubMed Central Homepage.* Nov. 2007. Environmental Health Perspectives. 25 Jan. 2009.
http://www.pubmedcentral.nih.gov/articlerender.fcgi?artid=2072855

Glamour Magazine[12] and on *Vanity Insanity*,[13] a Canadian TV series, describes the night she went to bed planning to kill herself the next day.

Kathryn got saline implants at the age of twenty-one. She grew up on the beach and augmenting her breasts to compliment her look in a bikini seemed natural to her. She recalls that having larger breasts boosted her self-image initially, and she loved having implants until she got sick. She developed symptoms after the birth of her first child.

She describes tingling sensations in her neck and arms, headaches, joint aches, chest pain that radiated down her left arm. She was breastfeeding her baby and developed thrush on her nipples. The baby also had a case of thrush in her mouth so severe that it caused bleeding. Kathryn saw several doctors, but they none of them could find a cause for her condition. She knew she was sick, but because she could not get medical confirmation of her illness, her friends and family started to doubt her. Even her husband, a busy law student at the time, began to suspect Kathryn's condition was "in her head."

She was, of course, devastated. She could find no help, no answers. No one understood. Besides being extremely ill, Kathryn was also completely alone. She was waging a very private battle for her life. Overwhelmed by the feeling that

---

[12] Cool, Lisa Collier. "Could Breast Implants Make You Sick?" *Glamour* Nov. 2000: 247-96.

[13] Bortolin, Ted and Barry Gray. "Vanity Insanity-Season 1; Episode 3." *Vanity Insanity*. Global TV. Burnaby, BC, Canada. 2006.

she was a burden to her family, she felt she could not go on. She made a decision to take an overdose of pills and end her life.

Thank goodness Kathryn decided to "sleep on it," because that night she dreamed that it was her breast implants that were causing her problems and that she should have them removed. The next morning, she got up and called a friend for advice. Her friend referred her to me.

Kathryn was suffering from a systemic fungal condition, plus a bacterial infection. When we removed her implants the saline solution inside was completely black, which is consistent with fungus. We sent the implants to Dr. Pierre Blais, the renowned Canadian chemist, for analysis, and he was so stunned by the amount of mold inside them that he personally called Kathryn and told her he just wanted to talk to the woman who had carried these implants inside her body. He understood that with that much mold in her implants, she had to have been very sick.

After treatment, Kathryn's condition improved quickly and now she leads a normal, healthy, productive life. She and her husband have another child and run a thriving business. Kathryn is committed to telling her story so that other women do not have to suffer the same fate she did. She believes now that a woman's self-esteem is derived from a healthy relationship with her body, that it is not physical beauty that inspires self-esteem, but physical health.

Kathryn's success story is not unusual. After treatment, these patients generally report that their mental and emotional states improve dramatically. Kathryn's "dark night of the soul" is not unusual either. Women routinely report that the psychological stress associated with breast implant disease is one of the most difficult and painful aspects of their conditions. These women relate horrifying stories of repeated misdiagnoses and the remarkable prevalence of doctors to dismiss their symptoms as imaginary because they are not able to establish a cause for their symptoms. Whether for physical or psychological reasons, suicide rates are significantly higher among women with breast implants.[14]

Looking back from the vantage point I now have, I understand why when I was guided to replace my silicone gel breast implants with saline implants, I was told by my internal guidance system, "It's not over yet." For my work, it was important to experience the illness and to understand its causes. Discovering the biotoxin connection to both saline and silicone breast implant disease has enabled me to offer effective treatment to yet another class of patients.

I notified the leadership of the plastic surgery society (as well as the ethics committee) of my findings, hoping that other doctors might benefit from my discoveries. The reception from these organizations was between apathy and hostility. Since I had seen quite a few patients who developed symptoms from sleeping on moldy mattresses after returning from hurricane evacuations, I contacted

---

[14] Fox, Maggie. "Breast Implants Linked with Suicide in Study." *Reuters.* 8 Aug. 2007. 25 Jan. 2009.
http://www.reuters.com/article/healthNews/idUSN0836919020070808?fe edType=RSS&rpc=22&sp=true

several plastic surgeons in Louisiana regarding this problem, and I was encouraged by their response. Even if the leadership within our societies is less than responsive to the need to educate plastic surgeons regarding this condition, at least some individual plastic surgeons in the communities affected by mold are listening.

PHOTOGRAPHS OF IMPLANTS

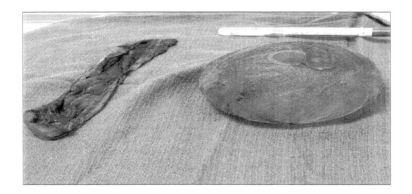

Intact Textured Silicone Implant with Capsule

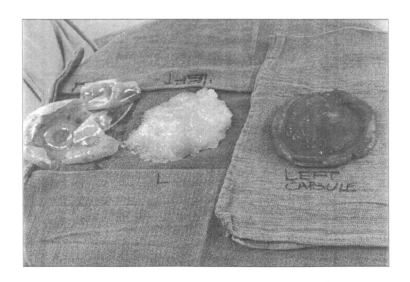

Ruptured Textured Silicone Implant with Capsule

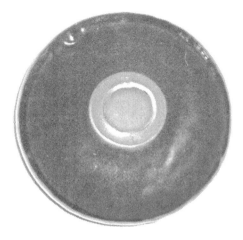

Smooth Saline Implant Discolored from Fungal Discoloration

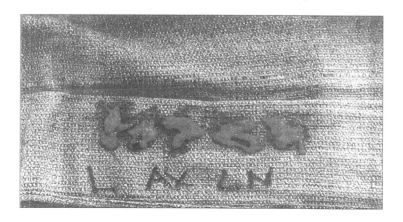

Axillary Lymph Nodes Filled with Silicone

SYMPTOMS OF SALINE IMPLANT DISEASE

SYMPTOMS OF SALINE IMPLANT DISEASE

Endocrine System

Thyroid:
- Hair loss
- Constipation
- Weight Gain
- Dry Skin
- Low basal metabolic temperature

ADH:
- Excessive thirst
- Shocks from static electricity
- Frequent urination

Adrenal:
- Low blood pressure
- Dizziness
- Passing out, especially with standing up quickly (orthostatic hypotension)
- Feeling as if you are dying

Sex Hormones:
- Irregular or lack of menses
- PMS
- Low Sex Drive

Neurological System

- Arrhythmias
- Cognitive Dysfunction
- Memory Loss
- Difficulty with Concentration
- Brain Fog
- Abnormal Brain MRI or Spectra Scan of the Brain
- Blurred Vision
- Sensory Loss
- Tingling
- Burning pain of extremities
- Muscle Weakness
- Balance Disturbance
- Burning Pain of the Chest Wall, Breast or Axilla
- Headaches
- Tremors
- Muscle Twitches
- Sharp pains
- Photosensitivity
- Seizures

Immune System

Viral Infections
- Mouth ulcers
- Herpes Simplex

Fungal Infections
- Chronic Urinary Tract Infections
- Mouth Ulcers
- Shortness of Breath
- Depression
- Fungal Rashes

Bacterial Infection
- Chronic Urinary Tract Infections
- Low grade fever
- Night Sweats
- Bronchitis
- Sinusitis
- Colitis
- Peridontal Disease

Autoimmune Disease (Intra-cellular bacteria) (Less common in bio-toxin patients)
- Rashes
- Joint Aches & Swelling
- Raynaud's Disease
- Dry eyes
- Dry mouth
- Difficulty Swallowing (less common than in silicone patients)
- Photosensitivity
- Abnormal Blood Clotting

Other Symptoms

- Muscle Aches
- Chronic Fatigue
- Lymph Node Enlargement
- Mal-absorption Syndrome
- Food Allergies

Heather's Story

Heather's story is remarkable in that she had worked as a scientist with FDA medical device regulations. She trusted that because the FDA had approved her saline implants, they must be safe, yet she nonetheless faced the medical complications they can cause.

Heather falls into a smaller category of patients who should avoid silicone in general. Certain HLA types such as HLA-B27 and HLA-DR 53 frequently develop autoimmune reactions if silicone is introduced into the body. Although some of her symptoms overlap with Pamela's symptoms, Pamela probably had a more classic biotoxin disease picture. Heather also had increased surgical bleeding which was treated during surgery with desmopressin. Within twenty minutes, her surgical bleeding was resolved. This alone, is reason enough to seek out services from an experienced explanting surgeon. Very few outpatient surgery centers stock this drug, which is so important in controlling excessive surgical bleeding.

"Getting breast implants has been the biggest mistake of my life, and I've made some pretty big mistakes. Prior to having children, I was lucky to fill out an A cup bra, but I never considered implants because I thought they were unnatural and risky. I was quite confident with my other personal characteristics. However, after nursing three children, I was left with very little breast tissue and my abdominal area was a wreck from the pregnancies.

"I'd gained the recommended 25-35 pounds with each pregnancy and lost the weight easily, but because I'm petite and do not have stretchy skin, I was left with a two inch gap between my abdominal muscles, an umbilical hernia, and disfigured skin that the term 'stretch marks' couldn't even begin to describe. When my husband and I knew our family was complete and I had weaned our last child from breastfeeding,

"I strongly considered the possibility of repairing my abdomen with a 'tummy tuck.' This was in the fall of 2004, when all the major networks had cosmetic makeover shows running during prime time. Women would get multiple cosmetic surgeries to completely transfigure themselves. Looking back, I was influenced by these shows in my consideration to add breast implants. Having the breast implant surgery so openly on television removed some of the taboo I held.

"When I told my husband I was thinking about breast implants, he was enthusiastic, but always said the decision was up to me. So I took my search to the Internet. I wasn't interested in newsgroups or chat rooms on the cosmetic procedures; I wanted to know what the FDA advised. I had previously worked as a scientist with

FDA medical device regulations, so I felt the FDA was the best authority when researching the risk of breast augmentation and abdominoplasty. The more I researched, the more I became comfortable with breast augmentation and saline implants, the 'safe implant.' I had more concerns about the risks associated with a tummy tuck procedure. My next step was finding a cosmetic surgeon.

"I only considered surgeons in my area and chose one that came recommended by friends who had both procedures prior and were happy with the results. The consultation appointment was booked two months out. This seemed like a long time to wait and my information packet instructed me to look at many Internet pictures of before and after breast augmentations to get an idea of what size implants I wanted. Looking at the Internet pictures,

"I thought that many of the women looked better in their before pictures than I would possibly hope to look in my after picture. I didn't want to have big breasts or get attention for their size; I just wanted to look normal. I decided that 300 cc implants would probably be a good size for me.

"The day of my consult finally came and I was very nervous. I had so many questions I wanted to ask the surgeon, and I forgot many. He was quick during my consult and talked me into 330 cc round smooth saline implants with an underarm incision site. We went over the risks very quickly. My biggest concerns were about the tummy tuck because the recovery time is much longer than for the breast augmentation. The surgeon assured me that I was young (early thirties), athletic, healthy, and would recovery quickly.

"At home, I reviewed the information with my husband and we made a decision to schedule the surgery. If I had the tummy tuck and the breast augmentation at the same time, we could save several thousand dollars in surgical and anesthesia fees, I would only have one recovery, and I would only need to arrange for childcare one time. What an efficient way to get my body back! My surgery was scheduled two months out, in March 2005, because that's what worked best with the childcare schedule.

"As the day approached, I became more convinced that my whole life would change with my new tummy and my new breasts. The only inkling I had that something might go wrong was while watching MTV's 'I Want a Famous Face.' The show featured young adults who had many plastic surgeries to look like someone famous, but in the middle of the show, MTV featured a negative story about cosmetic surgery.

"I specifically remember one where a young and healthy woman had breast implants and then her health deteriorated. She had her implants removed and her health improved, but she never fully recovered. Watching that segment, I felt panic. I immediately thought, 'The woman must be a hypochondriac, because the FDA has approved breast implants.' I went into my surgery with 99.9% confidence and a 'let's do this' attitude.

"It was the first surgery I'd ever had, so I was scared, but based on statistics, I was certain I would have a positive outcome. At first, I did. I woke up from surgery and had a serious pain in my chest from my muscles stretching. Over the next few days, I recovered in bed slowly. The tummy tuck healed well, but from the breast augmentation,

"I developed a cord on the right side of my underarm. I had to sleep on an incline for a few months and it also took about this amount of time for the cord to disappear. At that point I was very happy with how my breast implants looked and was a full B cup. Bra shopping was so much fun. My chest was less painful week by week, so I thought I was in the clear, but I was very wrong.

"It was May 2005, just two months after the surgery, and I noticed a lump on my middle right finger. I specifically noticed it because I used to wear a ring on that finger and it became difficult to take the ring on and off. My chiropractor looked at the bump and said that it was most likely a ganglion cyst. I stopped wearing my ring, but by the fall, the cyst had become so big it hurt when I bumped my right hand. I couldn't knock on doors.

"I saw my family practice doctor who examined the cyst, now very visible, purple and tender to the touch. He referred me to a hand surgeon. By the time I saw the hand surgeon after a two-month wait in November 2005, the cyst had grown so big and was so painful, I was wearing a metal cast around my finger.

"The hand surgeon diagnosed the cyst as a Giant Cell Tumor, and recommended surgery for removal. At home I researched Giant Cell Tumors and wanted to know if they were related to breast implants because in talking with a friend, I learned of women who developed rheumatoid arthritis after breast augmentation. I found no correlation between Giant Cell Tumors and breast implants, so I felt assured my implants were safe and not the cause of my new health problem.

"For insurance reasons, I had to wait two more

months for surgery, now my second surgery in my life. I was awake during the surgery because I only had a local anesthesia and heard the surgeon say he didn't think it was a Giant Cell Tumor, but a rheumatoid nodule. They also noted my hand turned blue during the surgery and asked if I had ever been diagnosed with Raynaud's phenomena. I had never heard of such a disorder.

"After the surgery, I began experiencing periods of my fingers turning white or blue when they were cold or hurt. This fit the symptoms of Raynaud's phenomena which was associated with rheumatoid arthritis. I saw the hand surgeon a few weeks later and received the results of the cyst biopsy. The pathology report revealed it in fact was a rheumatoid nodule. I asked him, 'Could this be from my breast implants?' He said that no, it couldn't, especially since my implants were saline, not silicone. In speaking with my family, I learned my grandmother had rheumatoid arthritis.

"Next, I saw my family physician with the results of my nodule biopsy and concerns about rheumatoid arthritis and breast implants. My physician assured me there was no connection between breast implants and autoimmune disease. He ran a Rheumatoid Factor test that came back negative. He convinced me the rheumatoid nodule was just a fluke and it was just a coincidence that it started two months after the breast augmentation. This was in February 2006, and I really wanted to believe him.

"The façade held up for a few months, and then everything came crashing down. In July 2006, I had appendicitis. This happens to 1 in 1,000 people. Certainly people without breast implants have appendicitis, but since the appendix is related to the immune system, I've often wondered if my implants could have been related to this. My appendix did not burst, but it was very close. I had several complications from the appendectomy surgery: atelectasis, abdominal hematoma, vertigo, bronchitis, walking pneumonia and superficial thrombophlebitis. Instead of the usual two weeks, it took me two months to recover from the surgery.

"Just when I was starting to feel like myself again in October 2006, the rheumatoid nodule came back on the middle right finger and another one started on my middle left finger. I went back to the hand surgeon. He said there was no point in operating, the nodules would keep coming back, I needed to see a rheumatologist and be put on autoimmune medications before my body destroyed my joints.

"Again I asked if my breast implant could have caused the nodule. This time, the hand surgeon said most studies found no causal relationship, but he knew several women whose autoimmune disorders improved after removing their breast implants. At this point, I was thinking, 'Please don't let it be true.' I'd only had my implants for a year and a half, so getting them removed was not at the top of my 'to do' list.

"I made an appointment with a rheumatologist, but I had to wait six weeks to get in. I started wearing braces on my hands. A vein protruded on one of my fingers and became very sensitive, so I had to cover that as well. Then I had an arthritis attack. My joints were painful in my fingers, thumbs, wrists, toes, ankles and my knees ached. I felt cold all the time, but my feet especially felt cold and wet. Even though they didn't feel cool to the touch, I wanted to sit in front of my space heater and warm up my hands and feet.

"The Raynaud's phenomena came back with a vengeance. I purchased arthritic gloves to keep my hands warm in the house and had to take extra precautions to keep my hands warm outside. The fatigue had become increasingly debilitating. At first I wasn't able to keep up with the housework, and I'd have to go to bed early. My husband did the extra housework on the evenings and weekends. Then the fatigue, combined with the joint pain, was so debilitating that I couldn't take care of my children as a full time mom. I had to get help from friends, neighbors and relatives.

"When I saw the rheumatologist in November 2006, I was at my worst. I was having trouble walking. He did a physical exam and ran forty different blood tests. Everything came back normal. The rheumatologist said the only explanation for my symptoms was my body was having a reaction to the breast implants and I should have them removed. Ironically, this was the same week the FDA approved silicone breast implants. I was stunned. How could the FDA approve the more dangerous silicone implants when my health had been destroyed by the 'safer' saline implants? Something was wrong with the picture.

"I started researching breast implant safety beyond the FDA's information. I joined a few Internet forums and learned of other women who had been through similar health experiences. These were the same women whom I'd previously written off as hypochondriacs. I read reports and articles on the potential conflicts of interest at the FDA and the breast implant manufacturers. Having a scientific background, I looked at the 'safety' studies in a new light and found that epidemiology could be manipulated to underestimate the autoimmune impact breast implants had on the health of some women.

"Now my mission was to get the implants removed, a breast explant. I learned from researching that not all cosmetic surgeons are qualified to perform this surgery and there are certain surgical methods that should be used, especially when the patient is ill. Based on lists of recommended surgeons kept by women who had previously been explanted, I would need to travel out of state. I didn't want to leave my children, so I went to my in-state cosmetic surgeon who performed my breast augmentation and tummy tuck.

"Before my appointment, my rheumatologist gave my cosmetic surgeon a call to explain my health situation and how it related to the implants. I knew he wasn't going to be my explant surgeon when he walked into the room and said, 'All you have in there is salt water.' I thought, first of all, this 'salt water' could be contaminated with bacteria, and second, these implants have a silicone shell. He offered his condolences several times and offered free surgical services for the explant. It was tempting, but I thought the method he would use was not safe. He was going to drain the 'salt water' through my original under arm incision, and then pull the implant. The capsule would be left intact. I thought this was not only dangerous because it would leave behind the toxin buildup in the capsule, but potentially expose me to the contamination in the saline.

"Next, I widened my surgeon search nationally. I quickly decided on Dr. Kolb in Atlanta, Georgia for several reasons. One was that she came highly recommended by several explant groups, but most importantly was she had a '*Silicone Immune Protocol*.' One of my family member's health had previously greatly improved on a heavy metal detoxification protocol, and I had spent a great deal of time researching the medical efficacy and safety of these protocols. Dr. Kolb's protocol shared many similarities to other protocols I had studied.

"In December 2006, I had my first appointment with Dr. Kolb and started on a portion of the protocol. Based on my insurance, the explant would be covered if medically necessary, and I had documentation from my rheumatologist and my internal medicine doctor that the surgery was necessary. Due to my childcare situation with out-of-state travel, I didn't schedule my explant surgery until March 2007. With the way I was feeling, three months would feel like three years, but I was able to greatly improve my health in those months just by making changes recommended by the protocol.

"I drastically changed my diet. I cut out dairy, wheat, chocolate, and nightshade foods (white potatoes, tomatoes, peppers). I added several vitamins and supplements to my daily routine: glucosamine, chondroitin, methylsulfonylmethane (MSM), Vitamin D3, Vitamin C complex, zinc, milk thistle, and acidophilus.

"My joint pain went from debilitating to manageable. The rheumatoid nodules in my fingers decreased. The fatigue decreased. I was still overtired most days and needed extra help with housework and was unable to participate in my usual outdoor activities. I just didn't have the energy. I would get cold easily, but I had enough energy to care for my children.

"The weeks dragged on during the three-month wait.

The one thing that was continually worse was breast pain. For several months I had a general uncomfortable feeling in my breasts. Some general and some specific, but a pinpoint spot developed where I had severe pain. Sometimes the pain prevented me from eating or sleeping.

"I scheduled a breast ultrasound exam at a local hospital's breast clinic. I didn't want a mammogram because of the small potential that the implant could be ruptured from the exam's pressure and since I was concerned about the saline contamination, this could be a recipe for disaster. When I checked in at the clinic, everything was normal. I was called back and told to change in a gown. Then I was lead into the mammogram room. I explained to the technician that I did not want a mammogram. I had scheduled an ultrasound and explained my reasons, showing her my referral and supporting studies. She said she'd consult the radiologist on staff.

"The radiologist refused to give me an ultrasound because it was out of their 'standard practice of care' and said that I might sue them if they missed something a mammogram would catch. However, I was insistent that I didn't want a mammogram and needed an ultrasound. To make a long story short, after going back and forth for two hours, I gave up. I was in tears as I changed back into my clothes to go home without an ultrasound.

"Just as I was about to leave, technician poked her head in the room and said I could have the ultrasound if I agreed to pay for it. They would not bill my insurance. Without much thought, I agreed. The ultrasound found five significant cysts. The cysts did not correspond to my severe pinpoint breast pain. If these had been seen on the mammogram, I would have needed the ultrasound anyway. Thankfully, my insurance was billed for the procedure.

"I have to admit, in the weeks leading up to the explant, I was an emotional mess. I couldn't wait to get rid of the implants, which had caused my health and body such pain and misery, but I was dreading having to go through the surgery and recovery. The prospect of returning to my pre-implant size did not bother me much. The week before the surgery, my internal medicine doctor prescribed an anti-anxiety medication for me. It was the only time I've take that type of prescription. I'm glad I did, because I was able to focus and get ready for my explant trip.

"My husband and I flew to Atlanta in March 2007; almost two years to the day of my breast implant surgery. On the first day, I had my consult with Dr. Kolb. It may have been different from many consults because I was 100% sure I wanted an explant and wanted Dr. Kolb to perform it. I had spoken with her on the phone several times before and corresponded many times through e-mail. I brought a big binder of previous tests, operative reports and contacts with me, and I handed them over to Dr. Kolb when I saw her. She highlighted that my symptoms were unusual. I had rheumatoid nodules and joint pain, but not rheumatoid arthritis. She recommended a test for the HLA-B27 antigen when I returned home.

"During the exam, she could externally feel the breast cysts and noted that one of my implants had dropped. After she pointed this out, I felt guilty that I hadn't noticed these things before. I think my implants were such a source of agony; I wanted to avoid them as much as possible for quite some time. Dr. Kolb planned to remove and biopsy the breast cysts during surgery. I filled my pre-surgery prescriptions that evening and prepared the hotel room for my after surgery care.

"The next morning was my preoperative physical. It involved basic testing, blood work, paper work and instructions. We went over the '*Silicone Immune Protocol*' and which supplements and vitamins I could add to help with detoxification. I added a few more. I felt like I was in a different world away from home, but I was certain I was on the path to healing. Finally the day of my explant arrived. It was scheduled for early in the morning.

"We arrived at the surgery center, my vitals were taken, and I was put under anesthesia. The next thing I remember, I woke up from surgery. This was the fourth surgery in my life, the first surgery being my breast implants. When I awoke, I asked for my husband and felt the severe pinpoint pain was even worse. My pain medication was increased. The recovery time at the surgery center was at least an hour longer than normal because I had a few surgery complications. I learned several things about myself.

"Overall, the explant was successful. The capsules and cysts were both removed and both being biopsied. Dr. Kolb thought I had a common benign condition called breast fibrocystic disease. On initial examination, my implants looked non-contaminated. The biggest issue was I bled a lot. Thankfully, during surgery I responded to a coagulant and stopped bleeding. Looking back at my medical history, I have always bled a lot; during previous surgeries, childbirth, dental procedures, but no medical professional had ever made issue of it. Dr. Kolb strongly recommended I be tested for a genetic bleeding disorder.

"After recovering at the center for two hours, I was able to get up with assistance. Amazingly, my breast pain was greatly improved. Dr. Kolb stated she did not see any physical reason why I had the pain and thought it was nerve compression. Thankfully, she was correct because within days of the surgery, the pinpoint pain was completely gone.

"Back at the hotel, the first day of recovery was rough. I was very weak from blood loss; my body retained all the fluids from the IV. I had a reaction to the antibiotic and a headache. My husband was essential in emptying the drains, helping me get in and out of bed and giving me medication. I had the pain pump, so there was not much pain from the explant.

"The next day was the postoperative visit with Dr. Kolb. Beyond the exam and instructions, we went over treatments options in case my symptoms did not improve in the next months. Finally, we flew home the next day. It was a long day home and even though I mostly used the handicapped services at the airport, I was very tired by the time I arrived home. It was so wonderful to see my kids. I felt like I had been gone for a month, but I had only been gone for four days.

"I had help with my children for the next week, and I needed it. I had my drains in at home for four days, and during that time I didn't leave my house, but rather rested as much as possible. It wasn't hard to stay put, as I was very tired from the blood loss. My husband easily removed my pain pump four days after surgery. Six days after surgery, my internal medicine doctor removed my drains. I couldn't wait to get home and get busy, but I wasn't so lucky.

"The next day one side had swelled up a bit, but with resting and icing, the swelling went down. I took it easy for another day. Now I was nine days past surgery and was amazed at how good I felt. My chest was sore, and I had to make sure my kids stayed away, but my joints felt better. I still was tired, but my iron was low and I was medically anemic, so I started on iron pills.

"Over the next month, things continued to improve. The rheumatoid nodule on my left hand completely went away, and on my right hand it appeared to be gone, but it was hard to say for sure because of the scar tissue from the surgery. The irritating vein on my finger was no longer present. I still was often tired and sometimes felt joint pain at night. When I was no longer required to wear the surgical binder, I went bra shopping. I bought the most heavily padded bras I'd ever seen and pads to sew into my swimsuit. In my opinion,

"I don't think anyone would notice that I had my breast implants removed when I wore my padded bras. Without my padded bras, I looked about the same as before the breast implants but with a little scar under each breast. My husband and I both agree that nothing is worth compromising my health.

"As I started to feel better, I started to 'cheat' on my diet. I added a little dairy here and a little wheat there. I didn't see any negative health effects and started eating more of my usual diet. Currently, I'm three and a half months past the explant surgery. I'm not as strict with my diet as I used to be, but I try to eat less dairy and wheat and no nightshade foods. I still take many supplements and vitamins daily. My joint pain is 99% gone. Every once and a while at night, I'll feel a little twinge of pain in my thumbs. I don't think I had that before implants. The breast pain from the implants is completely gone. The biopsies from the breast cysts came back benign.

"My implants were examined by a lab and found to have faulty valves and microbial contamination. I had an appointment with a hematologist. He was not able to find which genetic bleeding disorder I was affected by, but agreed I needed certain precautions during surgery. I tested positive for HLA-B27. After researching the topic and speaking with my family, I learned that 8% of the population is HLA-B27 positive. People with spondylitis are 95% HLA-B27 positive.

"My dad and grandpa have spondylitis, a type of arthritis. I had an appointment with my rheumatologist, but he was not able to relate how the finding fit together with my experience with implants. He said genetically, I have a 12% chance of developing spondylitis. I was offered several medications to treat a sub-clinical lupus disorder, but since I'm feeling better, I declined.

"The only problem that still plagues me is fatigue. It is miles better than when I was at my worst in November 2006, but I still don't have the energy I used to have. I feel like I'm getting better slowly. I've been told it can take six months to a year to get full improvement from the explant, so I'm hopeful my full energy will return. I'm able to take a few days to play and work like I used to, but then I pay for it. I'll be very tired for a few days. I have to work at pacing myself and not taking on too much. I often look in the mirror and see the dark circles under my eyes and think, 'I never used to have dark circles like that two years ago.'

"I wish I could say I wouldn't change this experience because I've learned so much about life and so much about myself, but I can't say that. There are many things I'd change. First off, I'd never get implants. I truly believe if I hadn't been inundated by cosmetic surgery shows, I would have not changed my long held views on breast implants. I truly believe I did not have access to adequate breast implant information because the FDA's and breast implant manufacturer's financial conflicts of interest affect the outcomes of their 'safety' and epidemiology studies.

"I truly believe I would have had my implants removed sooner had I not been mislead by several doctors on breast implant health risks. I've learned to completely document my family's medical history and research the possible adverse reactions or complications related to my history with all new medical procedures and medications. Medical professionals often overlook these issues.

"I've learned to be suspicious, but it's not a trait I wanted. Unfortunately, in today's medical world, it's necessary. I've also learned this is the only body I have and I have to take really good care of it because there are a lot of people who are depending on me. I'm going to have permanent health effects from breast implants. Thankfully, the effects have been minimized compared to what they could have been if I'd kept my implants longer or had them removed in an unsafe way. Like I said, getting breast implants has been the biggest mistake of my life."

-5-
RELATED TOXIC DISORDERS

"It has been appallingly obvious that our technology
has exceeded our humanity."
Albert Einstein

An unfortunate side effect of advancing technology is the
production of environmental toxins. Medical science cannot
keep pace in its understanding of the effect of toxic
substances on human physiology. Doctors (except for
environmental toxicologists) receive virtually no medical
education in the field of toxicology. And the current medical
literature (other than the toxicology literature) usually does
not address the potential for environmental toxins (both
chemical and biological) in the development of human
disease. Even if physicians have the insight to diagnose toxic

conditions, information on detoxification of the body from these chemical and biotoxins is not readily available to them in the standard medical literature. That is why I began to study holistic medicine, which addresses detoxification and functional medicine.

According to *Detoxification: A Clinical Monograph*, a report from the Institute for Functional Medicine, Inc., the process of detoxification involves several phases with multiple steps.[1] Factors that can affect the body's capacity to detoxify include a patient's general health, diet, lifestyle, age, gender, genetic factors and environmental factors, including the use of supplements and medications. I observed that once breast implant patients became ill, the problem of multiple chemical sensitivities was common and, in some cases, even progressed to electromagnetic sensitivity. In reviewing the literature on electromagnetic sensitivity, I discovered that increased numbers of free radicals are commonly found in these patients.[2] *In Detoxification: A Clinical Monograph*, the authors describe a number of common warning signs indicating chemical toxicity. These indicators include:

> ... a history of increasing sensitivity to exogenous exposures (toxic xenobiotics), abundant use of medications and

---

[1] *Detoxification: A Clinical Monograph*. Publication. Gig Harbor, WA: Institute for Functional Medicine, Inc., 1999: 1-42.
[2] Öckerman, Per-Arne. "Treating Electrosensitivity with *PAP IMI*." PAPIMI. 4 Aug. 1999. 25 Jan. 2009.
http://www.papimi.gr/cases/ockerman/ockerman2.htm

potentially toxic chemicals in the home or work environment *(or in the chest wall)*, sensitivity to odors and medications, musculoskeletal symptoms *(similar to fibromyalgia)*, cognitive dysfunction, unilateral paresthesia *(nerve symptoms)*, autonomic dysfunction and recurrent patterns of edema, worsening of symptoms after anesthesia or pregnancy, and paradoxical responses to medications or supplements. [3] (Italics mine).

I was seeing the same indicators in my patients with leaking breast implants.

My patients' systemic problems (fatigue, muscle aches, joint pain, vision and hearing impairment, etc.) were usually concurrent or closely related in time with chest wall symptoms (pain) and unilateral nerve symptoms (numbness on the side of the body with the leaking implant). This led me to the conclusion that they were suffering the effects of chemical toxicity originating from faulty breast implants. My own leaking Dow Corning Silastic II silicone gel implant led to localized chest wall symptoms on my left side only, including discomfort and burning pain which radiated down my left arm. I also experienced neurological symptoms including intermittent numbness on my left side. A neurologist later confirmed clinical evidence of left-sided thoracic outlet syndrome, probably due to inflammation around the brachial plexus from silicone in my lymphatic system. I not only observed the patterns of this disease in hundreds of patients, but also had the progressive disease

---

[3] *Detoxification: A Clinical Monograph*. Publication. Gig Harbor, WA: Institute for Functional Medicine, Inc., 1999: 1-42.

occurring in my body.

My detoxification protocols are based on information from monographs (such as the one mentioned above), input from holistic doctors from all over the country, observation of hundreds of similarly affected patients and experience of the progressive disease occurring in my own body. I have developed specific protocols for silicone toxicity, bio-toxicity, chemical and platinum toxicity.

(See http://www.plastikos.com for specific protocols.)

Each protocol begins by addressing a patient's diet to provide for nutritional healing. It recommends that the patient avoid foods that may be toxic or cause allergic reactions, which are common in these patients primarily due to yeast overgrowth in the gut. The protocols emphasize adequate clean water hydration to promote elimination of the toxins. We also recommend specific supplements that help in the biotransformation of toxins, effective treatment of inflammation, infections and endocrine imbalances. Because of my patient population, I was able to determine patterns of deficiency states, as well as which supplements were most effective for detoxification and immune support.

The detoxification organs in the body include the liver, the kidneys, the intestines and the skin. Most of the detoxification of chemicals occurs primarily in the liver and secondarily in the intestine. According to *Detoxification: A Clinical Monograph*, there are three systems involved in detoxification.[4] In phase one, detoxification enzymes such as cytochrome P450 system metabolize chemicals, especially in the liver. This process involves oxidation, reduction, hydrolysis, hydration and dehalogenation. Phase one processes can produce intermediate metabolites which can be toxic, including free radicals that have the ability to cause damage to proteins, DNA and RNA within the cell.[5]

Phase two processes take the reactive substances created from phase one, and through chemical reactions called conjugation reactions, the toxins are changed into relatively harmless and easily excreted substances. Phase two reactions require cofactors that are usually obtained from the diet, as well as energy in the form of ATP as produced by the Krebs cycle.[6]

The bottom line here is that if the body is attempting to detoxify many chemicals in the liver and the body's phase two system is not functioning properly, reactive substances produced in phase one are not neutralized in phase two. These toxic byproducts can cause significant intracellular damage and an increased risk of diseases, such as cancer and degenerative neurological disease. Peer-reviewed clinical studies show an increased risk of many cancers (excluding breast cancer) in patients with leaking or

---

[4] *Detoxification: A Clinical Monograph.* Publication. Gig Harbor, WA: Institute for Functional Medicine, Inc., 1999: 1-42.
[5] Ibid.
[6] Ibid.

ruptured silicone gel implants.[7] It is also interesting that neurological disease is one of the major categories in the Dow Corning settlement.[8] It could be that these diseases are related to a breakdown in phase two of the body's detoxification process caused by toxic overload.

The third phase of detoxification may be influenced by several systems such as gut microflora and alkalinity of the body, including the urine.[9] Diets and supplements that increase alkalinity (or pH) have positive clinical effects in most patients.

Silicone Toxicity

Silicone detoxification can be tricky because silicone gel is not a single substance but a collection of high molecular weight silicones with a smaller percentage of low molecular weight silicones. Although Dow Corning claimed that the high molecular weight silicones were inert, these substances have been shown to be able to modulate hormonal, endocrine and neurotransmitter functions.[10] In clinical studies, low molecular weight silicones have been shown to

---

[7] Brinton, L. A. and J. H. Lubin. "Cancer Risk at Sites Other Than the Breast Following Augmentation Mammoplasty." *Annals of Epidemiology* 11 (2001): 248-56.
[8] "Disease Claims." *Claimants' Advisory Committee.* 2008. 24 Jan. 2009 http://www.tortcomm.org/diseaseclaims.shtml
[9] *Detoxification: A Clinical Monograph.* Publication. Gig Harbor, WA: Institute for Functional Medicine, Inc., 1999: 1-42.
[10] Brawer, A. E. "Silicone and Matrix Macromolecules: New Research Opportunities for Old Diseases from Analysis of Potential Mechanisms of Breast Implant Toxicity." *Medical Hypotheses* 51 (1998): 27-35.

be widely distributed throughout the bodies of mice after a single subcutaneous injection.[11] Although it was believed that silicone could not be broken down in the body to silica, a biopsy of the sural nerve showed crystallized silicate in women with ruptured silicone gel breast implants.[12] Dr. Douglas Shanklin discovered that women with silicone gel implants excrete more silicate per day than women without implants. He suggested that inositol, a B vitamin, can promote the excretion of silicone from the body by converting silicone to silicate.[13] It is likely that the body's failure to eliminate these high molecular weight silicones contributes to the insidious illnesses seen in women once the silicone travels outside the Silastic envelope.

Chemical Toxicity

Chemical toxicity is found more frequently in patients with leaking silicone gel implants. It varies from patient to patient, depending on the genetic and environmental factors that influence the patient's ability to detoxify chemicals. I have seen elevated platinum levels in patients with saline

---

[11] Kala, Subbarao V., Ernest D. Lykissa, Matthew W. Neely, and Michael W. Lieberman. "Low Molecular Weight Silicones Are Widely Distributed after a Single Subcutaneous Injection in Mice." *American Journal of Pathology* 152 (1998): 645-49.

[12] United States Institute of Medicine. *Safety of Silicone Breast Implants.* Ed. Stuart Bondurant, Virginia Ernster, and Roger Herdman. Washington, DC: National Academy P, 1999: 247.

[13] Shanklin, Douglas. "Inositol." *Plastikos Plastic and Reconstructive Surgery.* 23 Feb. 2008. Millennium Healthcare. 19 Jan. 2009. http://plastikos.com/documents/Inositol.pdf

implants, although I am uncertain if platinum is still used as a catalyst. I believe that the implant companies have replaced platinum with tin. After placement of my Mentor smooth saline implants in 1997, serial hair analyses showed elevation of my tin levels. This elevated tin level gradually decreased over the subsequent years, probably due to my detoxification efforts. Chemical toxicity may also be related to the particular chemicals found in either the gel or the Silastic shell surrounding the gel and may vary according to the implant type and manufacturer. Chemical toxicity may also vary due to the total toxic load of the individual patient and may even involve interactions between the chemicals and/or silicone in the implant with other chemicals present in the patient's body from other sources.

Many of the chemicals listed as components of silicone gel implants are neurotoxins. This accounts for the extensive neurological component of the illness we see in women with ruptured or leaking silicone gel implants. Some of the chemicals are carcinogens, and this may account for the increased risk of certain cancers in this patient population. If one could obtain a specific chemical component list for each of the various types of implants, we would most likely see a correlation between the symptoms of the women and the material data safety sheet adverse effects data. Unfortunately, the FDA and the medical profession generally appear to have dismissed this data. The lesson learned should be to avoid putting these chemicals anywhere near an implant that is to be placed in the human body.

Patients ill from silicone gel implants not only suffer

from chemical toxicity from the implants, but they usually have a number of pharmaceutical agents in their systems, as well. Many poorly informed physicians prescribe drugs to treat misdiagnosed diseases such as serotonin related depression, irritable bowel syndrome, and autoimmune diseases such as lupus and multiple sclerosis. In addition, most women are on pain medication, anti-anxiety medication, muscle relaxants and sleep medication. These substances may only further overload the body's detoxification systems.

In my experience, the majority of patients experience depression, either as a result of having a chronic debilitating disease, or due to the effects of biotoxins from candidiasis or other fungi or mold. This produces a predictable chemical depression which is easily treated with anti-fungal therapy. Many of these patients do have symptoms of autoimmune disease, but it is an atypical connective tissue disease or an atypical neurological disease probably depending on the type of chemicals leaking out of the silicone gel implants.

A review of the list of chemicals found in silicone gel indicates that a number of the chemicals are toxic to the nerves. When physicians prescribe SSRI antidepressants for depression, which are not related to a serotonin deficiency, the patient's condition is likely to worsen. Some of these patients, commonly misdiagnosed with autoimmune diseases, have immune deficiencies. While investigators have discovered that immune cells are affected by serotonin, they don't yet understand exactly how.

Gerard Ahern, assistant professor of Pharmacology at Georgetown University and lead researcher on a study investigating the role of serotonin on immune response says, "The wider implication is that commonly used SSRI antidepressants, which target the uptake of serotonin into neurons, may also impact the uptake in immune cells."[14] Ahern concludes that SSRI's could have a beneficial effect on the immune systems of patients who are depressed and prone to infections, but it is also possible that such drugs could boost the immune system to the degree at which an autoimmune disease response is triggered. According to Ahern, "At this point we just don't know how these drugs might affect immunity, so we really need to clarify the normal role of serotonin in immune cell functioning."[15]

Among my patient population, I find that SSRI's further complicate the clinical picture. Unless the women were on SSRI's for a preexisting clinical depression, they usually feel better and their physical symptoms generally improve when they wean off their SSRI medication.

Another common misdiagnosis among the silicone immune disease population is a condition called irritable bowel syndrome. These patients do not actually have irritable bowel syndrome but rather dysbiosis, which is an overgrowth of unfriendly bacteria, yeast, and occasionally

---

[14] "SSRI antidepressants may also affect human immune system." *Medical News*. 23 Jan. 2006. 31 Jan. 2009.
http://www.news-medical.net/?id=15510
[15] Ibid.

THE NAKED TRUTH ABOUT BREAST IMPLANTS

parasites in the intestines.[16] This condition produces symptoms similar to irritable bowel syndrome (bloating, alternating diarrhea, constipation and abdominal discomfort) but the symptoms stem from a different source. When medications for irritable bowel syndrome are prescribed to patients who actually suffer from dysbiosis of the intestine, their symptoms may become worse. The overgrowth of unfriendly organisms is due to an immune deficit, and the condition improves with treatment of the immune problem. Treatment of the unfriendly bacteria, yeast, and in some cases, parasites is accomplished through the use of probiotics or friendly bacteria, antifungal agents, and supplements such as glutamine, which are effective in healing problems with leaky or impaired intestines.

According to the detoxification monograph, medicines such as the SSRI antidepressants and H2 blockers may inhibit one or more of the phase one enzyme systems.[17] In 1998, researchers published a study in the *Journal of the American Medical Association* entitled "Incidence of Adverse Drug Reactions in Hospitalized Patients," which reported that fatal adverse drug reactions may be much more common than previously realized and may be between the fourth and sixth leading cause of death in the United

---

[16] Koontz, D., J. Hinze, et al. "Leaky Gut Syndrome, Origins, Effects and Therapies, The Medical Link Between Dysbiosis and Many Major Ailments." *The Herbal Pharm* 19 (1999).

[17] *Detoxification: A Clinical Monograph.* Publication. Gig Harbor, WA: Institute for Functional Medicine, Inc., 1999: 1-42.

States.[18]

According to the detoxification monograph, "Accumulated data suggests that individuals with inhibited or compromised detoxification pathways would be more susceptible to adverse drug events."[19] The scientific study of these detoxification pathways indicate that many of the supplements suggested in the *Silicone Immune Protocol* are important for speeding up the phase two detoxification systems.[20]

Biotoxicity

Dr. Pierre Blais, a biochemist and biomaterials engineer and a former Senior Scientific Advisor to the Department of Health and Welfare in Canada, addresses biotoxicity in his paper "Residual Capsule and Intercapsular Debris as Long Term Risk Factors:"

> *Contamination of the space between the capsule and the implants by microorganisms, silicone oils, degradation products and gel impurities constitutes a major problem which potentiates the risk of implants. Such problems include inflammation, infection, deposition of mineral debris, as well as certain autoimmune phenomena. These*

---

[18] Lazarou, Jason, Bruce H. Pomeranz, and Paul N. Corey. "Incidence of Adverse Drug Reactions in Hospitalized Patients." *Journal of the American Medical Association* 279 (1998): 1200-1205.

[19] *Detoxification: A Clinical Monograph.* Publication. Gig Harbor, WA: Institute for Functional Medicine, Inc., 1999: 1-42.

[20] Kolb, Susan E. "The Silicone Immune Protocol" 2007. *Millennium Healthcare.* 19 Jan. 2009.
http://www.plastikos.com/documents/SiliconeImmuneProtocol.pdf

problems can be present when implants are in situ (in the body) and are often attributable to the implant. The logical expectation is that, upon removal of the implants, adverse effects will cease. This is an unjustifiably optimistic view. It is well documented from case histories that removal and/or replacement of implants without exhaustive debridement of the prosthetic site leads to failure and post surgical complications.[21]

At one time, it was assumed that removal of the fibrous capsule was not necessary, as it would "dissolve." A study reported in the *Plastic and Reconstructive Surgery Journal* states "Our findings show that the periprosthetic capsule may persist for at least 17 years after implant removal."[22] An earlier paper entitled "Complications Related to Retained Breast Implant Capsules" published in the same journal recommends total capsulectomy at the time of explantation, because implant capsules retained in the body:

> . . . *may result in a speculated mass suspicious for carcinoma, dense calcifications that obscure neighboring breast tissue on imaging studies, and cystic masses due to persistent serous effusion, expansile hematoma, or encapsulated silicone filled cysts. Retained capsules are a*

---

[21] Blais, Pierre. "Residual Capsule and Intercapsular Debris as Long Term Risk Factors." *Info-Implants Mammaires Inc.* 1997. 24 Jan. 2009. http://www.info-implants.com/Blais

[22] Rockwell, W. B., H. Casey, and Arthur Cheng. "Breast Implant Persistence after Breast Implant Removal." *Plastic and Reconstructive Surgery Journal* 101 (1998): 1085-088.

reservoir of retained foreign material.[23]

Total capsulectomy is often very tedious and time consuming, especially when 1) the implant was placed via the axillary approach with the capsule extending high into the chest wall and axilla, 2) when the implant was coated with polyurethane or is textured and the capsule is very vascular, 3) when the implant capsule is infected and is very inflamed, or 4) when the capsule is adherent to the chest wall and the surgeon can see the lungs expanding and contracting through the thin layer of tissue which remains between the chest cavity and the capsule.

Many surgeons will elect not to remove the capsule, as it is perceived to be less of an issue than the potential problems of chest wall perforation and pneumothorax (air in the chest cavity) due to this perforation. The problem with this decision is that the retained capsule acts as a reservoir for potential problems, including infection with bacteria, fungus and other atypical organisms.

Treatment is difficult, as these organisms enjoy a relatively walled off environment (scar tissue is difficult to reach with normal courses of antibiotics and antifungal agents). I have treated many patients with recurrent chest wall infections in which recovery is possible only after removal of the retained scar capsule.

---

[23] Hardt, N. S., L. Yu, G. LaTorre, and B. Steinbach. "Complications Related to Retained Breast Implant Capsules." *Plastic and Reconstructive Surgery Journal* 95 (1995): 364-71.

A more recent concept of biofilms (environments of microbial activity that form on the surfaces of implants) in the role of infections was introduced in a paper entitled "Biofilm in Implant Infections: Its Production and Regulation."

> *A significant proportion of medical implants become the focus of a device-related infection, difficult to eradicate because bacteria that cause these infections live in well-developed biofilms. Biofilm is a microbial derived sessile substratum or interface to each other, embedded in a matrix of extracellular polymeric substances that they have produced. Biofilm formation is partially controlled by quorum sensing, an interbacterial communication mechanism dependent on population density.[24]*

Biofilms may involve a variety of organisms: bacteria and fungi, as well as other pathogens. Unfortunately, the science of biomaterials and toxicology is largely absent from the medical education of most plastic surgeons. Frequently, the surgeons who implant these devices have never heard the terms biofilm or quorum sensing. Further, it is feasible that organisms, including fungi, may produce biotoxins that in very small amounts can cause significant illness in genetically susceptible individuals. These fungi may not be invasive into the healthy tissues, but tend to be present in the unhealthy scar tissue surrounding the implant or within

---

[24] Costerton, J. W., L. Montanaro, and C. R. Arciola. "Biofilm in Implant Infections: Its Production and Regulation." *International Journal of Artificial Organs* 28 (2005): 1062-1068.

the implants, especially the saline filled implants.

Platinum Toxicity

Chemical exposure, especially within the body, does not need to be in large doses to have detrimental effects. Researchers found platinum, which was used as a catalyst in the manufacturing process of some breast implants, to be the smoking gun, not just in women receiving the implants, but also in illnesses found in their children.[25,26]

These studies confirm what I have observed in my patient population: high platinum levels detected in hair analysis correlated with neurological and other symptoms of platinum toxicity, including severe allergies, asthma, nerve damage and decreased immune or autoimmune responses. Consequently, we developed a specific platinum detoxification protocol to assist patients in the elimination of this dangerous chemical toxin.[27]

The lesson in platinum toxicity is that it does not take much exposure to create disease. A paper published by Drs.

---

[25] Maharaj, S. V. and E. Lykissa. "Total Platinum in Urine of Women Exposed to Silicone Breast Implants and in their Children Conceived after Implantation by ICP-MS." *American Chemical Society Meeting.* Proc. of 230th National Meeting of the American Chemical Society Meeting, Washington, DC. Washington, DC: American Chemical Society, Aug. 28-Sept. 1 2005.
[26] Lykissa, E. D., and V. M. Maharaj. "Total Platinum Concentration and Platinum Oxidation States in Body Fluids, Tissue and Explants from Women Exposed to Silicone and Saline Breast Implants by IC-ICPMS." *Analytical Chemistry* 78 (2006): 2925-933.
[27] Kolb, Susan E., M.D. "Platinum Detox Protocol." 2008. *Millennium Healthcare.* 25 Jan. 2009.
http://www.plastikos.com/documents/PlatinumDetoxProgram.pdf

Lykissa and Maharaj in *Analytical Chemistry* in April 2006, proposed that the blood, urine and hair of eighteen of twenty-three women who had implants contained higher levels of platinum than the control group. In some of the women, they found evidence of platinum in oxidized reactive states, which are associated with toxic physiological effects.[28]

This paper, published by a widely respected scientific journal, became the center of a controversial debate over the role of platinum in illness from breast implants. *Analytical Chemistry* followed its publication of Lykissa and Maharaj's article with two letters from authors who represent the interests of the silicone implant manufacturers. Thomas Lane, a chemist at Dow Chemical, wrote one of the letters,[29] and Michael Brooks, who had testified before the FDA on behalf of Inamed Corporation in 2005, was the author of the other.[30] Both Lane and Brooks questioned Lykissa's research methods and interpretations.

Subsequently, the editors of *Analytical Chemistry*

---

[28] Lykissa, E. D., and V. M. Maharaj. "Total Platinum Concentration and Platinum Oxidation States in Body Fluids, Tissue and Explants from Women Exposed to Silicone and Saline Breast Implants by IC-ICPMS." *Analytical Chemistry* 78 (2006): 2925-933.

[29] Lane, Thomas H. "Comments on Total Platinum Concentration and Platinum Oxidation States in Body Fluids, Tissue, and Explants from Women Exposed to Silicone and Saline Breast Implants by IC-ICPMS." *Analytical Chemistry* 78 (2006): 5607-608.

[30] Brooks, Michael. "Comments on Total Platinum Concentration and Platinum Oxidation States in Body Fluids, Tissue, and Explants from Women Exposed to Silicone and Saline Breast Implants by IC-ICPMS." *Analytical Chemistry* 78 (2006): 5609-611.

issued an editorial warning stating that Lykissa and Maharaj's evidence flunked "this journal's standards."[31] One may wonder why *Analytical Chemistry* published the article in the first place if the research methods did not merit their approval. For an interesting editorial on this controversy, see "Platinum Bonds and Silicone Implants" on the *Acronym Required* website.[32] This article details the response to Lykissa's paper and suggests that controversial corporate interests may have played a role in *Analytical Chemistry*'s editorial decisions.

I find it extremely interesting that no further clinical studies were pursued when platinum levels in hair analysis were correlated with known toxic effects of platinum exposure in humans. In my opinion, this was because the two areas that the implant manufacturers most wanted to keep under wraps were platinum toxicity and the effect of platinum poisoning on children from exposure in utero or from breast feeding. If a solid link were established between breast implants and the devastating effects of platinum toxicity, it could ultimately cost the breast implant manufacturers far more in damages than did the silicone poisoning litigation.

---

[31] "Journal: Research Paper Probably Flawed." *PhysOrg.com*. 31 July 2006. 24 Jan. 2009.
http://www.physorg.com/news73578636.html
[32] "Silicone Implants Find Renewed Popularity in Market." *Acronym Required*. 16 Aug. 2006. 24 Jan. 2009.
http://acronymrequired.com/2006/08/platinum-bonds-and-silicone-im.html

Not only would the damages probably exceed those awarded to previous implant recipients, but an even higher settlement would likely go to their innocent children, many of whom suffer from significant neurological and immune system problems. Perhaps this is why, in spite of clear evidence to the contrary, a representative from Mentor Corporation said in an email to a reporter from *People Magazine*, "Platinum-related health problems in women with breast implants does not exist."[33]

A heartbreaking example of one woman's struggle with platinum poisoning is the story of P. J. Brent. She was the mother of seven children, five of whom were born before she got silicone breast implants. P.J. breast fed the two children born after she got implants. Subsequently, she and the two children developed symptoms associated with platinum toxicity: joint pain, fatigue, gastrointestinal distress and neurological symptoms. One of her children was eventually confined to a wheel chair.

In 2000, P.J. testified before the FDA about the devastating health effects she suffered as a result of her silicone breast implants. Two months later she "allegedly" jumped to her death from a parking deck at an Atlanta shopping mall. An autopsy found platinum in her heart, lungs and brain. Her husband quotes the pathologist who performed the autopsy as saying, "A woman with that much platinum in her brain could not have been thinking

---

[33] Adato, Allison, Susan Schneider Simison, and Melody Simmons. "The Return of Silicone?" *People* 63 (2 May 2005): 81-84.

rationally." Mr. Brent attributed her suicide to the guilt she felt because she believed she had caused her children's health problems.[34]

The Precautionary Principle is a concept that has been broadly applied internationally to address conflicts in science, medicine, the environment and law. It simply states: *"If it is within our power, we have an ethical imperative to prevent rather than merely to treat disease, even in the face of scientific uncertainty."*[35]

This concept, which is expressed in a number of international treaties and applied by a variety of policy making bodies throughout the world, can be seen as the evolution of the idea contained in the ancient medical principle, "First, do no harm." It also reflects common sense adages such as "look before you leap," "better safe than sorry" and "an ounce of prevention is worth a pound of cure." If the conflicting research over the safety of breast implants is a case of scientific uncertainly, then shouldn't the FDA and other regulatory institutions err on the side of caution? Shouldn't breast implants be withheld from the market until they are proven safe? As the authors of the Acronym Required article state:

---

[34] Hanes, Allison. "In the Bosom of Death: Suicide Risk Is High among Breast Implant Recipients, Canadian Study Says." *National Post* [Don Mills, Ontario, Canada] 11 Oct. 2006: A22.

[35] Raffensperger, Carolyn. "Precautionary Principle: Bearing Witness to and Alleviating Suffering," *Environmental Research Foundation*. 22 Jan. 2003. 24 Jan. 2009 http://www.rachel.org/en/node/5625

So while it seems that neither the FDA nor the journal can really judge the veracity of competing conclusions in the available research, both the journal and the FDA nonetheless appear to favor the opinions of scientists with vested interests in promoting implants. The FDA has repeatedly discounted Lykissa's work. Yet he is not the only scientist with these concerns. Where are the "neutral" scientists? After a quarter of a century, women are still confronted with a sea of confusing, biased data in the leaky boat that is the science research on silicone implants.[36]

I suggest that neutral scientific research in this area no longer exists, because the scientists who express any interest in clinical trials at universities are simply not supported or are actively suppressed. A nonprofit group dedicated to fighting the use of silicone implants sponsored Lykissa's latest research. Given the editorial response from *Analytical Chemistry* (who, after all, believed the research was good enough to publish in the first place), it is also evident to me that the journals may not be immune from outside influences. As the article in *Acronym Required* questions:

The journal didn't accommodate a rebuttal from the original authors when they published Lane's and Brook's critiques. Should we trust that the science was lousy? Or should we wonder whether the journal was swayed by the critics' affiliations with Dow Corning Corporation, Mentor

---

[36] "Silicone Implants Find Renewed Popularity in Market." *Acronym Required.* 16 Aug. 2006. 24 Jan. 2009
http://acronymrequired.com/2006/08/platinum-bonds-and-silicone-im.html

Corporation, and Inamed Corporation?[37]

Nonetheless, the medical lesson from the platinum issue is clear. The body changes even small amounts of potentially toxic substances found in implants into reactive intermediates that can be very dangerous. Because this condition is seen in my patient population, I specifically look for platinum toxicity and if present, recommend a platinum detoxification program.

Morgellons Disease

Morgellons disease is a devastating condition that may be caused by a combination of chemical and biological agents reacting with the systems of the body. The symptoms include persistent skin lesions that are associated with fiber-like filaments, granules and crystals that appear under the skin or protrude through the skin lesions, infection, debilitating fatigue, joint and muscle pain and mental fog. Morgellons patients often suffer from the sensation that insects are crawling under their skin. For this reason, their condition is often misdiagnosed as delusional parasitosis. These parasites have been documented.

The medical establishment has denied the existence of Morgellons Disease and marginalized its sufferers as

---

[37] "Silicone Implants Find Renewed Popularity in Market." *Acronym Required.* 16 Aug. 2006. 24 Jan. 2009.
http://acronymrequired.com/2006/08/platinum-bonds-and-silicone-im.html

psychologically disturbed, accusing them of faking their symptoms to get attention. However, due to the mounting clinical evidence, the United States Center for Disease Control created a task force to study the condition.[38] In 2008, the CDC launched a study with Kaiser Permanente's Northern California Division of Research to investigate the increasing number of cases in the Bay area.[39]

A possible explanation for the high incidence of Morgellons disease in patients with silicone implant disease is the possible combination of implant related chemicals with chemicals in the food supply. This connection is suggested in a paper presented by Dr. Hildegarde Staninger. She reports, *"Toxicological pathology identification of tissue biopsies from an individual diagnosed with Morgellons revealed the presence of continual silica or glass tubules with the presence of silicone."*[40]

A private study to determine the composition of Morgellons fibers has determined that the fibers' outer

---

[38] Stobe, Mike. "CDC Probes Bizarre Morgellons Condition." *CBS News - Breaking News Headlines: Business, Entertainment & World News.* 9 Aug. 2006. 24 Jan. 2009.
http://www.cbsnews.com/stories/2006/08/09/ap/health/mainD8JCII281.shtml

[39] United States Center for Disease Control and Prevention. "CDC to Launch Study on Unexplained Illness." Press release. *Center for Disease Control and Prevention.* 16 Jan. 2008. 24 Jan. 2009.
http://www.cdc.gov/media/pressrel/2008/r080116.htm

[40] Karjoo, Rahim, and Hildegarde Staninger. "Toxicological Pathology Evaluation of Tissue Biopsy Specimens of a Morgellon Patient." *American College of Pathology* (Pending publication).

casing is made up of high-density polyethylene fiber.[41] Dr. Staninger reports that this material is used in the bio-nanotechnology world as a compound to encapsulate a viral protein envelope that is sprayed on food such as luncheon meat in order to prevent Listeria infections. This viral cocktail contains six different viruses intended to prevent Listeria bacterial infections, which can infect food such as deli meat.

Food manufacturers began spraying this viral cocktail on meats and vegetables in August of 2006.[42] Unfortunately for patients already exposed to silicone, there are no labeling requirements for these viral phages, so it is difficult to know which foods to avoid. Several of my patients with previous silicone exposure developed an exacerbation of their Morgellons disease after eating luncheon meat frequently *in the last quarter of 2006.*

The problem of producing multiple fibers (which come out of their bodies) improved when these patients discontinued eating luncheon meats. This could be indicative of what may occur when chemicals foreign to the human body interact with each other inside the body. Such chemical interactions may affect the systems of the body in ways that we cannot predict and could contribute to new

---

[41] Staninger, Hildegarde. *Fiber Made of High Density Polyethylene* (HDPE). Laboratory report. Lakewood, CA: Integrative Health International, LLC, 2006.
[42] "Staninger Interview." Temple of Health Radion Program. Telephone Interview. 2 Aug. 2008.

disease states.

The quest to determine if silicone exposure causes a particular problem in every patient may too simplistic. There are many patient variations, including consideration of other toxic exposures, as well as the rate at which the patient is able to detoxify chemicals. Unfortunately, silicone is not only one chemical, but a "chemical soup." Implants produced by various manufacturers or at different times can include a variety of chemical compositions, depending on the specific implant.

Finally, there are different types of toxicities to consider. Silicone toxicity has an autoimmune basis in some patients, saline related toxicity involves a biotoxin from mold contamination, and others may involve chemical toxicity from a combination of different sources. To complicate matters further, the effect of several of these toxicities may be delayed for eight to fifteen years due to the lifespan of the Silastic shell surrounding the silicone gel.

Raynaud's Disease

Another known chemical in silicone gel is methyl ethyl ketone. The toxic effects of this compound are associated with Raynaud's disease, which is present in many of my patients with silicone gel breast implant disease. Raynaud's disease occurs because of a vascular problem of the extremities, which results in a lack of circulation. If the loss of circulation is severe enough, it can cause sores or tissue loss on the digits of the hands or feet.

We need to be much more careful about chemicals placed in the body. Not only is there potential for biological systems to be affected by these chemicals, but in some cases, chemicals may interact inside the body and change into far more dangerous intermediates.

I recently treated a patient who suffered from a severe case of Raynaud's disease. He had so much tissue loss on three fingertips on his right hand that the bones were exposed. He had also had an amputation of a portion of his left index finger. This particular patient had been to various medical specialists, and none of them could determine a cause for the disease or help him with his progressive symptoms. He had been referred to a pain clinic for pain control, but their specialists had nothing to offer other than pain medication.

After listening to the patient's story, my guidance was to ask him a specific question. "Have you been handling any chemicals preceding the onset of your illness?" He immediately replied that he had used methyl ethyl ketone without gloves in the year prior to the onset of Raynaud's symptoms. The chemical exposure had involved specific contact with his damaged fingers, so I pulled out and showed him my list of chemicals found in silicone gel implants. Methyl ethyl ketone was the first chemical on the list and silicone patients frequently had Raynaud's disease.

I started him on a chemical detoxification protocol and referred him to an environmental toxicologist, because Raynaud's disease is not the only problem this chemical can cause. He was amazed that a plastic surgeon would so quickly pinpoint the cause of his problem. Without the correct diagnosis, the treatment of this disease is very difficult.

When I asked Dr. Staninger how methyl ethyl ketone could cause Raynaud's disease, she replied that it was via depletion of amino acids. I was then able to locate a paper on the success of oral arginine in the treatment of Reynaud's with digital necrosis.[43] With chemical detoxification as well as arginine replacement we were able to treat his Raynaud's disease and successfully complete the surgery to remove and cover the exposed bones at his fingertips.

Immune Disorders

In an article entitled "Pathogenic and Diagnostic Aspects of Siliconosis," published in *Reviews on Environmental Health* in 2002, Drs. Shanklin and Smalley reviewed the chemistry and the immunopathology of siliconosis.[44] They discussed the potential effects of siloxanes (found in contraceptive devices and personal care products, as well as in some medications such as antacids) on the body. Siliconosis is defined as an immunopathic process within the body (created by exposure to silicone) "with a potential to induce or stimulate autoimmune states over a long-term, beyond its evident capacity to induce chronic inflammation, granulomas and fibrosis."[45]

---

[43] Rembold, Christopher and Carlos Ayers. "Oral L-Arginine Can Reverse Digital Necrosis in Raynaud's Phenomenon." *Molecular and Cellular Biochemistry* 244 (2003): 139-41.

[44] Shanklin, D. R. and D. L. Smalley. "Pathogenic and Diagnostic Aspects of Siliconosis." *Reviews on Environmental Health* 17 (2002): 85-105.

[45] Shanklin, D. R. and D. L. Smalley. "The Immunopathology of Siliconosis: History, Clinical Presentation, and Relation to Silicosis and the Chemistry of Silicon and Silicone." *Immunologic Research* 18 (1998): 125-73.

Many of my patients experience a silicone disease symptom flare when they start using a cleaning or personal care product that contains silicone. Silicone's chemical structure allows it to readily enter the skin upon contact, so they are again exposed to agents that can cause their disease to flare. When they stop the exposure and start the detoxification program again, their symptoms improve.

Autoimmune disorders can occur due to silicone and chemical exposure in susceptible individuals. Autoimmune disorders can also develop because of the longstanding immune problems brought about by chemical and biotoxin exposure, which is characterized by a natural killer T cell deficiency and sometimes a white cell deficiency. These patients have evidence of an intracellular mycoplasma infection and usually develop a clinical picture that more resembles scleroderma and rheumatoid arthritis than the usual picture of atypical connective tissue disease.

Treatment of this infection consists of the immune protocol and long term antibiotics (that are not cell wall dependent), along with antifungals to prevent fungal overgrowth. It is also important to rule out intracellular spirochete infections (such as Lyme disease) and systemic viral infections (such as HHV6 and CMV) as these are common in the immune compromised individual and need specific treatment as well.

Generally, toxic exposure disrupts the immune system and makes the individual more susceptible to those autoimmune diseases that are characterized by intracellular infective agents. Some chemicals may directly stimulate an autoimmune effect in genetically susceptible patients.

Janice R.'s Story

Janice's story demonstrates how a silicone induced immune deficit makes some women susceptible to other life-threatening illnesses. After many years of searching, including visits to fifty-four different doctors, Janice finally received an accurate diagnosis of her condition and began treatment. She was suffering from Morgellons disease and Lyme disease, in addition to silicone immune disease and atypical neurological disease from her implant complications.

From the infectious disease specialist at Johns Hopkins (who recommended psychiatric treatment) to the dermatologist at another prominent medical center (who diagnosed Janice with delusional parasitosis), the medical profession repeatedly failed Janice. She is truly one of those patients who has been disowned and ousted by the traditional medical system due to its inability to recognize when a patient is ill, and in Janice's case, critically ill.

Janice has done a remarkable job of recording her

illness with photographs taken over a series of years. They could provide a wealth of information for any researcher interested in studying this disease. Her cognitive dysfunction, which is sometimes is quite severe, is due to an organic brain injury resulting from the effects of silicone and Morgellons disease. Even though abnormal brain MRI images indicated this problem, many doctors still failed to diagnose it.

Her spirit and tenacity to seek out those who are experts in their respective fields has probably saved her life. In the early 1990s, I was given a vision of Plastikos Surgery Center, and at this time I was told that the center would be built "for the disasters." I would come to learn that the meaning of "the disasters" was patients who had been ousted from the traditional medical system. Despite being severely ill, they were not able to find help anywhere else.

The patients in this category require a combination of traditional and holistic medicine, as well as intuitive guidance to determine protocols on which to base their treatment. Janice is one example. Treating Janice and other silicone patients who have developed Morgellons disease gave me opportunity to develop a protocol to treat this disease, as well.

"I had breast implant surgery in 1985 and had no problems with them whatsoever for sixteen years. My health was fine, and at 43-years-old, I was on top of the world. In fact, my dreams were all finally coming true.

"My life, thus far, had been a colorful journey. I was gifted as a child with the ability to paint anything I looked at. I spent the better part of 25 years pursuing my dream to become an artist, painting 12 to 18 hours a day and producing a large volume of images. The majority of my work was of ethnic cultures in their traditional garb, spiritual paintings and angels. I had the ability to tap into universal power and actually channel the images I painted. At a very young age, I began interacting with the angelic kingdom. In today's terms, I guess I'd be considered an indigo child. I used my art for years to battle many addictions and problems that I had. I escaped into my art.

"Because I painted to live rather than lived to paint, I had never learned to market my art, as it was necessary for me to focus on paying my bills at the end of the month. Yet I realized that I was doing what I loved and believed that one day I would be recognized for it. Finally, I landed a big break. In May of 2001, my art was scheduled for publication by one of the best art publishers in the country. I breathed a sigh of relief. My art would finally be out there and the world would see the color and the healing power it possessed. I believed I was doing the work God put me on this planet to do.

"At the time, I was working as a traveling sales representative for an art publisher and was covering three states. I was making more money in a month than I had made in previous years as an artist. One day I was visiting an account I'd called on many times before, and I had a very strange experience. For some reason, something went wrong in my brain and I got very disoriented. I didn't recognize anything in my surroundings. I forgot why I was there. Nothing like this had ever happened to me before, and it was extremely distressing. In fact, I was so distraught that I wasn't able to go back to my job after that.

"I was also having back pain at the time, but it never occurred to me that it might be related to this mental lapse, so I went to a psychiatrist thinking that the source of my condition must be mental. He ran tests and diagnosed me with severe attention deficit disorder and anxiety disorder. He prescribed medications for both conditions.

"Shortly after that, I began to lose feeling in my hands, and soon I wasn't able to use them. This, of course, increased my anxiety tremendously because I could no longer paint, and that was incredibly scary for me. I went from doctor to doctor trying to find out what was going on, but no one could help me. One doctor tested me for heavy metals and found that I had high levels of metals in my body, but I knew there was so much more going on than that. My whole body ached. I spent thousands of dollars on massage, chiropractic treatment and acupuncture, but nothing was working, and my health continued to deteriorate.

"I wondered if my implants could be causing these problems. Since 1997, I had suspected that one of them was ruptured. My breasts had started to change shape. The right breast had become much smaller and had started to push underneath my armpit. I had several mammograms, ultrasounds and MRI's, and each one showed a protrusion of some sort, always indicating a need for more tests. More tests were done, but no one ever felt it was necessary to follow up further than testing. I contacted the doctor who implanted me, and he had mysteriously lost my file.

"I called my brother who is a board certified plastic surgeon and asked his advice. He assured me that the controversy surrounding breast implants was all media hype and that there was no such thing as silicone sickness. He told me I was just having a midlife crisis and that it had nothing to do with my implants. I went to several other plastic surgeons, and they each said I was fine, though they never looked at any of my tests.

"Meanwhile, my symptoms continued to get worse. I got a severe neurological tic, I could barely walk and I developed a horrible shake and tremor in my neck. Most of the time I was in such a mental stupor that I had no idea what was going on around me. I had appointments with toxicologists, neurologists and plastic surgeons, anyone I thought might be able to help me.

"I was desperate to find answers, but when I described my symptoms, I found most doctors refused to take me seriously. I was shocked and horrified by the way I was treated. Every doctor I went to said there was nothing wrong with me. Many thought I was delusional. I saw some of the finest doctors in the country and most of them thought I was simply nuts. The doctors would come into the room, never really look at my tests and never look at my body. Apparently, they thought I was a hysterical woman who only believed she had ruptured implants.

"One doctor diagnosed me with fibrocystic disease and sent me home to take vitamin E. I later found out that my brother, the plastic surgeon, had been calling ahead of me, telling doctors before I got there that I was dealing with a midlife crisis and that they should just appease me and send me on my way.

"By August of 2001, I still had no answers, but I had a

complete armory of medications: uppers, downers, pills to wake me up, pills to put me to sleep, pills for pain, pills for concentration, pills for depression and pills for anxiety. I knew I had to be explanted, and after much searching, I finally found a doctor who agreed to do it. While I was waiting in his office to schedule the surgery, his nurse came in and said, 'You might want to do it early in the morning because he starts to drink.' I decided to find another doctor.

"One day I was in my garden, and I got down on my knees and started to pray. I begged God to please, please help me get these implants out. I needed to get my brain working, I needed my hands back and I needed to resume my life. Out of the blue, the former producer of a controversial radio program that I was on for two years gave me a phone call. He needed someone to sit in that day and act as a co-host, and later that day I was on the air.

"The host opened the show by saying, 'Did you ever try to get a doctor's appointment and have to wait like six weeks to see someone?' Well, that was my ticket. I appealed my case to the listening audience. I said, 'I have a problem. I have a ruptured silicone breast implant and I've seen 15 doctors to date and no one will take them out.' Within minutes a plastic surgeon called in and offered to help. Two weeks later, I was in the operating room.

"The doctor who took my silicone implants out told me I had to replace them with saline implants. He told me I wouldn't be able to handle the condition of my breasts after explant surgery and that the new implants were perfectly safe. So he took out my silicone implants that day and replaced them with saline implants.

"The day after the surgery, I was covered with skin lesions and burns from head to toe. I had them all over face, my abdomen and my chest. When I showed the doctor these sores, he left the room came back with three nurses. He looked at my mother and said he had done what he could do for me but that I was a self-mutilator and suggested that I see a psychiatrist. This crushed me. I knew something was very, very wrong with this picture. The medical reports from my surgery stated that no silicone rupture was found, even though the surgeon had told me he had to chisel my chest cavity for an hour and a half to get all the silicone out. He told me he had never seen anything like it, that it was hardened on my ribs.

"By this time, I knew about Dr. Kolb's practice, because I had spent hours on the Internet researching silicone sickness. I called her office and told her what I had been going through. When I told her my doctor had told me I was self-mutilating, she said, 'Honey, those are toxic wounds from exposure to the chemicals in your body. You're OK. You're not a self-mutilator. Just relax. You'll start to heal and everything will be fine.'

"Unfortunately, this turned out to be just the beginning of a long nightmare. The lesions never stopped, and instead they started to get increasingly intense. I ended up going to an integrative physician in Philadelphia. My mother would pack me into the back of her car and drive two and a half hours to take me to this doctor. I thought he was going to be my savior. He was using chelation therapy and IV vitamin bags to try to detoxify the chemicals from my body.

"It was during this time that I started seeing worms

and fibers coming through my skin. I showed these things to the doctor, and he indicated that he believed me. For me, having parasites did not seem all that far-fetched. I had spent a great deal of time traveling around the world. I'd been to a lot of third world regions, which didn't have the most sanitary conditions.

"Meanwhile, I was still seeing the psychiatrist, and he continued to increase the amount of drugs I was using. By the time I was finished with him, I was on medication for attention deficit disorder, depression, pain and insomnia. As a result, I was in a stupor most of the time. I couldn't get out of bed. My brain was like a piece of mush. I couldn't think for myself; I couldn't speak for myself. I lost the ability to walk. I was scared because I wasn't getting any answers, and I wasn't getting any better. Instead I was getting worse.

"I had no explanation for all kinds of weird and horrifying things that were coming out of my body. Worms were coming out of my ears; fibrous strands were emerging through sores in my skin. At the same time, my brother was on a campaign to turn my family against me, saying I was making my illness up to get attention. I wanted people to know I wasn't crazy. I felt that I needed to prove that I was sick, so I started to document this illness as it progressed through my body. I started to take photographs of what was happening to me.

"Near the end of 2003, both my psychiatrist and my integrative doctor turned me away. Even though I had spent over $67,000 on alternative treatments and thousands more on visits to the psychiatrist, the two doctors had consulted with each other and decided I was nuts. Apparently, neither of them believed that my photographs were authentic.

"By this time, I was having complications from my new saline implants. I had had them in my chest for nine months and there was no doubt in my mind that my body was rejecting them. I went back to the doctor who took out my silicone implants, even though he had called me a self-mutilator. I was clear that I needed to get those things out, and he was the only doctor available at that time to do it.

"When I found several lumps in my breasts in the spring of 2004, I decided to travel to Atlanta to see Dr. Kolb. I was so sick I could hardly get out of bed and could barely walk. After ten minutes in her office, I breathed a sigh of relief. It was the first time in years I felt comfortable with a doctor. Everything I told her my body was going through, she assured me was from the implants. She assured me that I wasn't nuts, that I was among the Silicone Sick and that my experience was not only real, but also shared by thousands of women throughout the world.

"She ran a barrage of tests and told me I was a candidate for surgery. She went in and removed twelve lumps and, by the grace of God, none of them were cancerous. Due to my impaired immune function, however, I developed infections from the surgery and got very sick. Even so, I felt great because I was finally in the hands of a capable doctor, someone I could trust. I was confident Dr. Kolb was going to find a way I could get well again.

"I made nine trips to Atlanta over the course of the next three years, and I was always impressed with the quality of her care. She managed to work me into her busy schedule at a moment's notice, and no matter if there were fifteen other patients in her waiting room, she would spend as much time as necessary with me. She listened intently to the lists of ailments I presented her with. No matter what time of day or night, through email or by phone, she was always there and always willing to listen and help. I got so much peace as a result of her presence in my life. This is a very scary illness and it gave me great comfort to know that she not only believed me, but also understood what I was going through.

"Dr. Kolb suggested I go to visit Dr. Arthur Brawer, a rheumatologist familiar with silicone sickness, as she believed he could tell me more about what was going on with me. When I got there, I showed Dr. Brawer my photographs and finally, I got some relief. Dr. Brawer showed me photographs of other patients who had lesions similar to mine. He told me that what I was experiencing was not atypical of someone who goes through silicone sickness.

"My illness was progressing rapidly, and I felt I was dying. Worms were coming out of sores on my body. Threads, fibers, hard balls, black specks and all these creepy things were coming out of my skin. I was terribly sick, confined to my bed and alone in my house while this was going on. To make matters far, far worse, almost nobody believed me. By this time, my brother, the plastic surgeon, had even turned my family against me saying I was doing all this for attention. My parents were wavering because my brother was telling them that I was nuts, but right there in front of them, they could see that I was literally dying. The only person I knew who believed me was Dr. Kolb.

"I finally got an appointment at Johns Hopkins Hospital, hoping that a team of doctors there would research my case and find the answers I needed. I took 29 vials of parasite samples, my collection of photographs and a movie that showed a live worm in my blood cell analysis. But when the doctors came in, they never even examined me. They looked at my pictures and accused me of taking the pictures off the Internet. They wrote up a seven-page report saying I was schizophrenic, bipolar and had refused psychiatric treatment. They tried to lock me up in a mental institute that day.

"Next Dr. Kolb suggested I find a specialist to treat my digestive problems. In 2005, I found Dr. Trent Nichols. I went to see him with my little vials of worms and all my pictures. He looked at me and said something I had never heard before. He said, 'You've got Morgellons disease.' I'd had already had several brain MRI's which showed I had lesions in my frontal lobe, but no one could determine why. Dr. Nichols told me that brain lesions like mine were associated with Morgellons disease. He also tested me for Lyme disease and the test came back positive.

"It was great to finally have some kind of diagnosis, but there was still no cure for my illness, and no one knew anything about it or what to do about it. I came back home and spent days and days and days in bed not able to get out, not able to function, not able to walk, not able to talk, not able to remember what I did five minutes before. My hands still didn't work, and my legs weren't working. All I wanted to do was get well so I could get back to my life and get back to my art. At this point I wasn't even sure I was going to be able to keep my house. It really, really got bad.

"I went to various doctors trying to find a cure, and finally found Dr. James Overman, who specialized in the treatment of parasites, in Ohio. I sent samples of the parasites I had collected to him, and several days later, he called me. He wanted me to come to Ohio so he could examine me.

"After my initial consultation with Dr. Overman, he told me he couldn't understand how I was still alive. I had extensive parasite damage to my skin, ranging from holes where insects had come out, to rashes, scars, bumps, depressions, swellings, twisted hairs and patches with very little hairs. The normal shape of my ears was distorted by parasite damage, both eardrums were scarred, and I had lost 50% of my hearing. I had parasite damage to both eyes and both sides of my head were completely bald.

"By this time I was 47 years old, and I had been extremely ill for five years, fighting against a horrible debilitating disease that the medical community refused to acknowledge. The rupture of my silicone breast implants five years earlier had marked the onset of a nightmarish descent into illness. Because of the effect the silicone had on my immune system, I had become susceptible to all sorts of other problems. Besides having worms coming out of my skin, I had been bedridden most of the time and had a tendency toward loss of balance and slurred speech. My hands were numb, making it impossible for me to work. Worst of all, I couldn't paint.

"One thing I want to emphasize is that the stress, fear, sadness and isolation of someone who is chronically ill is just beyond the comprehension of a healthy person. I always thought that when someone got sick, you went to their side. But when someone is sick for years, people forget about them and abandon them. People should not turn their backs on someone who is ill. I've been fighting a very scary, very lonely battle.

"Another extremely difficult aspect of my illness was the fear that I might be contagious. With all this stuff coming off of me and falling out of me, worms, larva and so on, it was always in the back of my head that everywhere I walked, I might be leaving something behind that could spread to other people. This was very scary. To date, however, it does not appear that Morgellons disease is something that can be passed along from person to person. Dr. Kolb tells me that the latest research indicates it's a vector borne illness. So at least I have some peace in my heart now, knowing that I'm not infecting anybody.

"I've also had to deal with the extreme financial burden my illness has created, not only for me, but also for my mother. I've had to file bankruptcy, and I've had my car repossessed. My mother had to mortgage her house when she was 79 years old. We've had to cash in all stocks and insurance policies. My treatment still runs about $2,000 per month. The Catholic Church paid for my last visit to Atlanta to see Dr. Kolb. There are days I go without food and water. At times I've had to sell possessions just to get something to eat. I keep thinking today will be the day I can go back to work and straighten this out, but so far, that day has not come. Just as soon as I start to feel better, I get whacked with something else due to my compromised immune system.

"I take some comfort in the role I played in helping to determine a cause and a treatment protocol for Morgellons disease. If I can save someone from the horror

I have experienced through telling my story, then perhaps my suffering will not have been in vain. I know there are others like me who are searching for answers and being told their problems are psychological. I am here to say that Morgellons disease is a very real condition. In my search for answers, I went to 54 doctors and, in spite of the physical evidence I presented them with, 99% of those doctors wrote in my file that I was nuts.

"What I had was severe brain impairment, probably caused by the effects of parasites, yet most doctors I saw believed I was delusional. I have fought very, very hard to stay alive and to get this word out to people. I hope all the research and all the documentation I've done helps humanity on some level because that's why we're here. We're here to help our fellow man and to learn new things in science and to keep growing as a people.

"The biggest lesson I've learned is that the medical community is not there to find answers. If your symptoms don't fit neatly into their little box, into one of their pre-established categories, or if you don't have a condition they already know how to diagnose and treat, you're not going to get any help. If you're suffering from something they don't understand and don't already have a diagnosis for, then most doctors aren't equipped to help you find a solution.

"When confronted with something they don't understand, they react with fear and disbelief. If they don't understand what is happening in your body, they prefer to believe that it isn't real. Even some of the naturopaths I saw were so frustrated by what was going on with my body that they too got scared and turned me away.

"The difference between Dr. Kolb and many other

doctors is that she listens without judgment. She goes above and beyond the call of duty because she is a true healer. When I started to present with worms, sores and weird things coming out of my body, she never hesitated to reach out and hug me. I found this very comforting, even remarkable considering we didn't know whether I was contagious or not at that time. She literally holds her patients hands. She has the capacity to love without fear. During the black plague, the doctors who wanted to work as healers stayed, and the ones who were afraid ran for their lives. I have tremendous respect for her brilliance, but even more for her compassion. She is truly an amazing doctor and woman.

"I am frustrated that most of western medicine still fails to acknowledge my illness. I recently made an appointment with a dermatologist at Hershey Medical Center because I want mainstream medicine to understand this parasitic infestation. I walked in with all my information, but when I said Morgellons, they chuckled. The doctors at Hershey Medical Center told me I was suffering from delusional parasitosis. They diagnosed my condition as acne. Instead of getting angry, this time I just walked away with sadness. Morgellons disease affects thousands of people, and doctors aren't able to treat it. That is sad.

"I was recently diagnosed with cancer in my brain and liver, and have started natural and homeopathic treatments. I still have sores and things coming though my skin. I've started to regain some of the use of my hands and my neurological damage is starting to reverse due to the herbal programs I'm on. I eat only organic foods, free range meats and have to stick to a very alkaline diet.

"The Lyme disease was in remission for a while, but now it has kicked back up again. I have days where I'm out of bed and functioning at about 50%, and then there are days where I can't do anything at all. My heart is big, and my hope and my faith are huge. I trust that God will give us the answer one day for a cure. I also pray for the ability to educate people not only about Morgellons, but also about silicone sickness because it is a very ugly journey."

-6-
DETOXIFICATION PROTOCOLS

"Those who say it cannot be done should not get
in the way of those doing it."
Chinese proverb

Detoxification essentially refers to the removal of foreign substances from the body through the natural processes of elimination. We come in contact with a multitude of environmental toxins through the food we eat, the air we breathe, the water we drink and the chemicals we are exposed to every day, but our natural defenses protect us in most cases. If, by chance, small amounts of toxins penetrate our defenses, our bodies have natural mechanisms to get rid of them.

Our body breaks down toxins so that we can eliminate them through our skin, blood, lungs, liver, kidneys and intestines. This process involves the biotransformation of chemicals or molecules that are foreign to the body into excretable metabolites. If the body accumulates toxins in amounts larger than the elimination systems can process, then illness can occur. In Breast Implant Disease we see the ravages wrought by chemical as well as biotoxicity.

According to *Detoxification: A Clinical Monograph*[1] from the Institute for Functional Medicine, Inc., the majority of detoxification occurs in the liver and a smaller amount in the intestinal mucosal wall. The monograph describes in detail two phases of the detoxification process. Phase One involves the P450 cytochrome system and other enzyme systems that produce reactive intermediates, including free radicals. Phase Two involves conjugation reactions including a requirement for sufficient glutathione and the requirement for cofactors, which are dependent on ATP production. After these conjugation reactions, the chemical becomes more hydrophilic (water loving) and can be eliminated in the urine or bile.

Deficiencies within the Phase Two system (which may be due to deficiencies of glutathione, amino acids such as glycine or methyl donor groups such as MSM and SAMe) may result in a build up of reactive intermediates, including free radicals that can cause secondary tissue damage and predispose the patient to cancer. Thus, without careful monitoring during both phases, the detoxification process

---

[1] *Detoxification: A Clinical Monograph*. Publication. Gig Harbor, WA: Institute for Functional Medicine, Inc., 1999: 1-42.

can go awry and cause more harm than good.

Factors that influence detoxification activity include genetics, age, gender, disease, health status (particularly involving diseases of the liver), diet, lifestyle and the effect of medications. According to *Detoxification: A Clinical Monograph*, when the system is overwhelmed by chemicals (and silicone when breast implants start to leak or rupture), the clinical presentation of toxicity includes:

> ...a history of increasing sensitivity to exogenous exposures, sensitivity to odors and medications, musculoskeletal symptoms (similar to fibromyalgia), cognitive dysfunction, unilateral paresthesia, autonomic dysfunction in recurrent patterns of edema, and paradoxical responses to medications or supplements.[2]

As these are the most common symptoms of silicone immune disease, it made sense to develop detoxification protocols to help women suffering from this condition. *The Silicone Immune Protocol* was originally designed using the principles outlined in this monograph and has been developed over time through a program of continued research and clinical observation.[3]

The protocol includes support for all the body's elimination systems, and nutritional support is provided

---

[2] *Detoxification: A Clinical Monograph*. Publication. Gig Harbor, WA: Institute for Functional Medicine, Inc., 1999: 1-42.

[3] Kolb, Susan E. "The Silicone Immune Protocol" 2007. *Millennium Healthcare*. 19 Jan. 2009.
http://www.plastikos.com/documents/SiliconeImmuneProtocol.pdf

through a detoxification diet and supplements. We recommend foods with nutrients that function as cofactors (required in the biotransformation process) and eliminate foods that are likely to contain toxins, food allergens and substances that increase cytokines and other inflammatory substances. We emphasize adequate hydration with clean water. We supply supplements to assist Phase Two reactions (during which biotransformation molecules are conjugated).

The protocol supports gastrointestinal health, including integrity of the gut mucosa, because the proper balance of intestinal microflora is critical in detoxification. Pathogenic bacteria in the intestines can produce toxins that leak through the intestinal wall and increase toxicity throughout the body causing a condition known as leaky gut syndrome. Gut microflora can also produce substances that can either inhibit or increase detoxification. The balance of gut microflora is supported, as well, through diet and supplements.

Another important factor in detoxification is the body's acid-alkaline status. Overall, a slightly alkaline state in the body induces detoxification. Alkalinity is influenced by diet, water and supplements designed to increase alkalinity (such as Buffer pH™).

Silicone and Chemical Detoxification

Patients with silicone poisoning respond to treatment using the *Silicone Immune Protocol* and their conditions improve. They have less fatigue and mental clouding, fewer muscle aches, less chronic infections and periodontal disease, less dizziness and neurological symptoms (such as numbness of the extremities) and less chest wall discomfort. Joint pain and rashes also improve as the chemicals are eliminated from the body. In general, patients who have had longer exposure to the silicone and chemicals due to prolonged leakage and/or rupture of the breast implants require a less aggressive detoxification approach. Their systems are much more fragile due to their increased toxic load.

In patients with significant heavy metal and chemical exposure, tailored detoxification programs are designed after data is collected from tests such as Toxic Hair Analysis and other laboratory data. Based on the patient's unique clinical situation, which is evaluated during a history, physical examination and pertinent laboratory tests, an individual and highly specific detoxification protocol is designed. Each patient receives an additional immune support protocol to enable her to withstand surgery without complications such as infection.

In some cases, the detoxification and immune protocols alone are not sufficient for the patient to regain her health. Sometimes surgery to remove retained silicone in the breast, chest wall, axilla, lymph nodes or capsules is necessary.

Immune function improves with supplements that increase natural killer T cells and other glyconutrients, thymic factors and transfer factors. Patients whose immune functions are not supported in the perioperative period have increased incidences of infection in the postoperative period. Supplements to support liver detoxification, heavy metal detoxification, chemical detoxification and silicone detoxification are also provided in the protocol. Dr. Douglas Shanklin found that inositol, a B vitamin, helps the body eliminate silicone. By increasing its conversion to silicate, it can be eliminated in the urine.[4] Supplements and herbal products that support liver detoxification, as well as Phase Two of intracellular detoxification, are also used.

Biotoxin Detoxification

Biotoxin detoxification requires the elimination of the bacteria, virus, fungus or parasite that is producing the toxic reaction in the body. The most common biotoxins that produce significant symptoms in breast implant patients are from yeast or mold, both of which are classified as fungi. Surgery may be necessary to eliminate organisms that live in the protected scar capsule, because such environments are resistant to anti-fungal and antibiotic therapy.

Most often the patients experience relief of the symptoms while on antifungal treatment, but when the treatment is discontinued, the symptoms rapidly recur. After the capsule or infected lymph node is surgically removed, their symptoms generally clear up. This is in alignment with the surgical principle that an infected foreign body is resistant to drug treatment alone and requires removal of the foreign body to resolve the symptoms. Once the source of the biotoxin had been found and eliminated from the patient's body, as well as from her

---

[4] Shanklin, Douglas. "Inositol." 23 Feb. 2008. *Millennium Healthcare*. 19 Jan. 2009.
http://plastikos.com/documents/Inositol.pdf

environment, detoxification of the biotoxin can be accomplished.

Biotoxins are small molecules that are hydrophobic (i.e., dislike water and like lipids, such as lipids found in cell wall membranes) so that they tend to be tightly attached to cell walls. They particularly like the cell walls of myelin sheaths, which is why biotoxins most often function as neurotoxins. Biotoxins cannot be directly measured, but their effects can be measured with either a visual contrast sensitivity test or an alpha MSH laboratory test.

Biotoxin detoxification is accomplished with herbal supplements, butyrate (which helps dislodge the biotoxin from the cell wall), supplements that increased intracellular glutathione and fibers that bind the biotoxin in the intestines.

Platinum Detoxification

For women who were exposed to breast implants in which platinum was used as a catalyst in the manufacturing process rather than tin, we developed an additional Platinum Detoxification Protocol.[5]

Platinum levels are most easily followed from a hair analysis test although other testing methods such as urine and nail analysis may be used. Platinum levels should also be checked in children who were in utero or breast fed by

---

[5] Kolb, Susan E. "Platinum Detox Protocol." 2008. *Millennium Healthcare.* 25 Jan. 2009.
http://www.plastikos.com/documents/PlatinumDetoxProgram.pdf

women who were ill or who had ruptured or leaking silicone implants, especially if the mothers have high platinum levels on hair analysis testing.

Morgellons Disease Protocol

An additional protocol for Morgellons disease was developed to treat silicone and saline breast implant patients who also developed this condition.[6] Morgellons patients often have a preexisting condition that has contributed to an immune deficiency. Besides a high incidence of patients with prior silicone exposure from breast implants, I also see women who have had prior chemotherapy treatment, Lyme disease or mold exposure who are now suffering from Morgellons disease. These patients have an extensive infected foreign body not just of the skin, but also of the organs including the neurological system and brain.

In treating Morgellons disease, we use supplements to address the immune deficit, as well as the underlying infections. The infections can be viral, bacterial (including intracellular infections), fungal, parasitic and arthropod infestations. The detoxification programs to treat this condition are designed to help remove the foreign body, which may be a fiber network of silicone and polycarbonates. Extensive detoxification programs and

---

[6] Kolb, Susan E. "Morgellons Disease Protocol." 2008a. *Millennium Healthcare*. 25 Jan. 2009.
http://www.plastikos.com/documents/MorgellonsDiseaseProtocol.pdf

significant antioxidants are needed for these patients to improve. This is a life threatening illness that, if left untreated, may render patients unable to care for themselves. Morgellons patients are sometimes prone to suicide due to feelings of hopelessness and despair. It is a devastating condition made worse by the lack of appropriate attention and care from most of the medical profession.

An important part of the treatment protocol involves attention to cleaning the patient's environment, as re-infection from the debris created by Morgellons disease is common. The fibers protruding from the lesions are not just in the skin, but deeper, as well, and are infected. The patient's surroundings can become contaminated from "shedding" fibers, and these fibers seem to be able to re-infect the patient.

Morgellons Disease has only recently been recognized by the United States Center for Disease Control.[7] The head of the Morgellons team of the CDC saw her first patient with the disease in my clinic, and since then, only slight progress has been made in the research of its cause and treatment. While the Morgellons Protocol has helped patients to regain a portion of their health, more specific information about the origins of this debilitating disease is needed.

---

[7] United States. Center for Disease Control and Prevention. "Unexplained Dermopathy (aka Morgellons." *Center for Disease Control.* 16 Jan. 2008. 24 Jan. 2009.
http://www.cdc.gov/unexplaineddermopathy/general_info.html

Cynthia's Story

Cynthia's story emphasizes the danger of massage around the area of damaged silicone breast implants. Many patients described exacerbations after massage therapy. After having a massage, Cynthia developed serious pain and inflammation on her right side, associated with pain in her right shoulder. Eventually, she developed frozen shoulder.

Even though these symptoms occurred on her right side, during Cynthia's explant surgery, I found that she had a more extensive rupture of her left silicone implant. I learned from Cynthia what I had suspected in other patients: specifically that it is *infection* of the foreign material caused by the defective implant that is associated with unilateral frozen shoulder.

The synchronicity of Cynthia working as the aesthetician in my clinic at the time her body broke down shows us that if we trust our guidance, we can be led where we need to be for the help we do not yet know we need to receive.

"After working for years as an aesthetician in the beauty industry, I began seeking a job in medical aesthetics. It had always been my heart's desire to work in the medical field as an aesthetician. Little did I know that my desire would lead me to the 'right place at the right time.' The following paragraphs are the story of my journey that led me to Dr. Susan Kolb and the consequences I suffered due to silicone breast implants.

"In the late 80s, I began contemplating having a breast augmentation. I wanted bigger breasts because I was always very small-chested and I wanted to look nicer in bathing suits and lingerie. I seemed out of proportion and it really affected my confidence. I thought that having bigger breasts would boost my self-assurance. My husband and I discussed the matter, and I decided to begin a search for a trusted plastic surgeon. Through many consultations with other women who had previously had the surgery, I finally decided on a particular surgeon and made my mind up to follow through with my mission.

"During the consultation with my surgeon, my husband and I were led to believe that the implants that I would be receiving would be saline. We had heard of the controversy surrounding silicone implants and had made the decision that we wanted to go with the saline implants. Our surgeon also informed me that the implants would last at least twenty years. It was not until many years later that I discovered that my implants were silicone and not saline.

"My close friend at the time was having a breast augmentation with the same surgeon. She, too, was under the impression that the implants that she would be receiving were saline. It was not until my yearly check up with my surgeon seven or eight years later that he informed me that I had silicone breast implants. He told me not to be alarmed and that the controversy surrounding silicone implants had no scientific basis. He assured me that silicone would in no way do my body harm, even if there was to be some leakage from the implants.

"Approximately fifteen years after the breast augmentation, I went for my yearly checkup appointment with the same surgeon. When I told him that my implants had hardened, he did not advise me to have them removed or replaced. He only told me that if I was comfortable, then they were fine. I remember leaving his office feeling somewhat uncomfortable with the cold and impersonal treatment I had received. This was very typical behavior of the doctor, so I brushed it off as not being a major issue.

"As time went by, I started having problems with my arms feeling numb and having pain in my right shoulder. I thought that these were ergonomic problems due to my job as an aesthetician.

"Being the spiritual person that I am, I began asking God to lead me and direct me to a new job in the medical field of aesthetics. One day as I was browsing through a website looking for work, I ran across an advertisement for a position as an aesthetician at Plastikos Plastic and Reconstructive Surgery. After a couple of interviews, I was hired for the position. I believed that God had directed my path there for a reason.

"I had only been working for Dr. Kolb for about three months, when the pain that I had previously been experiencing worsened. Not knowing exactly what to do, I went for numerous massage therapy sessions. After one particular session, I was in so much pain that it felt as though I had been hit in the chest and back with a baseball bat.

"My husband was so concerned that he wanted me to go to the hospital and make sure that I had not had some sort of injury. We went to the emergency room, where they did numerous tests and took x-rays. The doctors at the hospital knew that I had implants, but they could not find anything wrong with me. They sent me home with pain medication.

"In the following days, I conveyed to Dr. Kolb what I was experiencing and asked her if the pain I was experiencing could possibly be related to my implants. After examining me, she concluded that not only were my implants probably leaking, they were very infected and that was what was causing the pain and inflammation. You could actually feel the heat resonating from my body. Dr. Kolb prescribed anti-inflammatory medicine and antibiotics. She also told me to start the silicone immune protocol that she had designed that consisted of a strict diet of mostly fish and vegetables and numerous supplements. On many occasions, Dr. Kolb took time out of her busy day to perform healings for my shoulder. The pain subsided enough for me to work and carry out my normal duties as an aesthetician. Aestheticians use a lot upper body motion, which was where my pain was.

"After a month of going through the 'red tape' of getting insurance approval for surgery, I finally had my implants removed. The surgery was five hours of tedious labor for Dr. Kolb, as she removed the implants and free silicone from my body. After the surgery, Dr. Kolb told me that my left implant had probably been ruptured for several years. My right implant had not been ruptured for as long as the left implant. The pain in my shoulder still remained and resulted in a frozen shoulder.

"It has been two years since my explant surgery, and I am feeling much better. I am experiencing no more pain and I have almost all my range of motion. The surgery left me with my left breast smaller than my right one because Dr. Kolb had to remove more tissue affected by the silicone leakage. She counseled and informed me that I should not receive new implants until the infection was completely cleared up, which more than likely would be six months post surgery.

"Until this day, I have been indecisive as to whether to opt for another breast augmentation. I have learned to look at myself nude in the mirror and completely love who I am, even with disfigured breasts. This is one of the many spiritual lessons that I learned through this experience. I do not define who I am by my outward appearance. God loves me for who I am and because I have a heart towards Him. My confidence is my relationship with God and not about how perfect my body can be. Of course, this does not mean that I won't have a breast augmentation again, but I will certainly be a different person than I was before.

"I believe that everything happens for a reason. Looking back, I know that God directed me to apply for the position with Dr. Kolb's practice. I was in the perfect place to receive the care I needed for this particular journey in my life. I learned to listen to my inner voice. That voice told me something was wrong with my implants."

-7-
SPIRITUAL MEANING OF DISEASE

"The only real valuable thing is intuition."
Albert Einstein

Esoteric teachings throughout history emphasize a common, universal principle. This principle is stated succinctly as "as above, so below." First found in The Emerald Tablets of Hermes Trismegistus, a legendary text outlining the quest and attainment of an Egyptian priest and sage, this concept has to do with the relationship between the macrocosm and the microcosm.[1] It indicates that what transpires in the higher realms of existence will naturally be reflected in the physical world and vice versa. The physical, emotional,

---

[1] Hauck, Dennis William. *The Emerald Tablet: Alchemy of Personal Transformation.* New York: Putnam Penguin Books, 1999.

mental and spiritual realms are intricately related, bound in a universal web and, in essence, cannot be separated. All things are independent, yet interrelated: mind and body, atom and galaxy, the individual and the collective. All exist together in a holographic universe in which everything is connected, and each of the parts mirrors the sum of the whole. It may be further stated that, according to this principle, the thoughts and beliefs we hold in our consciousness are manifested in our third dimensional reality.

This principle predicts that the toxic problems of the collective mind will be reflected in toxic diseases manifesting in the human population. It is no secret that we are facing a critical time in our history and that our future as a species hangs in a precarious balance. Human activity is even affecting the weather of the planet as global warming looms ominously before us, threatening our very survival.

Our advancing technologies bring with them unsuspected dangers. With the advent of microwaves, cell phones, computers and other electronic mechanisms, we are exposed to new forms of radiation, which may be dangerous to our health. We ingest pesticides, plastics, genetically engineered organisms, chemically treated water and genetically modified foods without understanding the effects they may have on our bodies. Our dependency on fossil fuels and our addiction to consumption is reaching crisis proportions as we cloud the air we breathe with CO_2 emissions and pollute our oceans, river and streams with chemicals from manufacturing.

As we go through life, we are exposed to a variety of

heavy metals and plastics of all sorts: from the lining of aluminum cans to those present in IV catheters. We introduce foreign substances into our bodies through dental amalgams, implants, internal prosthetic devices, suture material left within the body, tattoos, hair pigments and personal care products such as shampoos, conditioners, deodorants and antiperspirants, after-shave lotions, perfumes and cosmetics, residue from dry cleaning, food additives and drugs and their break down products. Also, consider the chemical contamination of our food, air and water sources.

I wonder just how much foreign material is introduced into the human body over a lifetime and how much the body can stand. The common theory is that the cumulative effect of these toxins leads to the free radical formation that is associated with disease, immune-related deficiencies and accelerated aging.

Our bodies have natural detoxification and elimination systems to handle much of this load. However, biochemical analysis of the majority of people in industrialized societies shows high levels of many substances including aluminum, mercury, lead and other heavy metals.[2] It is well established that toxic overload in the bowels can lead to "leaky gut" syndrome and allow large molecules to enter the body and produce autoimmune reactions that may affect the joints

---

[2] United States Center for Disease Control and Prevention. *Third National Report on Human Exposure to Environmental Chemicals.* Rep. Atlanta, GA: Center for Disease Control and Prevention, 2005.

and other tissues.[3] Given the rapid reversal of joint aches
and conditions such as bursitis after the removal of leaking
silicone gel implants, and knowing that silicone acts as an
adjuvant in the immune system, I feel that we have much to
learn regarding the mechanisms of autoimmune disease in
relationship to these foreign substances.

The Gulf War syndrome is another example of
technology gone awry. It is possible that the chemical agent
"squalene" acts as an adjuvant to initiate this condition. A
genetically modified intracellular mycoplasma may also be a
factor in this disease.[4] The Gulf War syndrome has many
characteristics similar to silicone immune dysfunction,
including not only autoimmune, but also the neurological
symptoms. Could these foreign materials that we introduce
to our bodies through vaccines, implants, prostheses and
ingestion of contaminated food and water be contributing to
the epidemic of autoimmune diseases that we are seeing in
our society?

It is not what we know, but what we do not know about
the effect of the multitude of chemicals, plastics, metals,
drugs and their metabolites to which we expose our bodies
that concerns me. What are the effects on enzyme systems,

---

[3] Koontz, D., J. Hinze, and Et al. "Leaky Gut Syndrome, Origins, Effects
and Therapies, The Medical Link Between Dysbiosis and Many Major
Ailments." *The Herbal Pharm* 19 (1999).

[4] Nicolson, Garth L., Nancy L. Nicolson, and Marwan Nasralla.
"Mycoplasmal Infections and Fibromyalgia/Chronic Fatigue Illness (Gulf
War Illness) Associated with Deployment to Operation Desert Storm."
International Journal of Medicine 1 (1998): 80-92.

cell membranes and our DNA? What are the effects on interference with repair mechanisms and on mitochondria energy production? What are the effects of the emerging field of nanotechnology which has introduced substances into our food and personal care products without the requirement of labeling and for which there is little research regarding the long-term toxic effects of these unique substances?

No wonder we currently have epidemics of energy disorders such as fibromyalgia, chronic fatigue syndrome and atypical autoimmune diseases, which evade traditional medical understanding. A healthy immune system cannot exist if foreign chemicals, heavy metals and nutritional deficiencies are constantly bombarding it.

The good news is that advanced therapeutic methods exist to eliminate the free radicals and detoxify the body of a number of chemicals, heavy metals and other contaminants within the body. Detoxification programs, including chelation therapy, removal of mercury amalgams and restoration of gut intestinal flora with elimination of pathogenic flora, are standard treatments of cancer in Europe.

Other detoxification programs include diet, nutritional supplements, fasting, far infrared heat, massage, hydrotherapy, yoga, exercise, sauna treatments, magnetic clay extraction packs, colon, liver, kidney and gastrointestinal tract cleanses, colonics and lymph stimulation and ionic and electrolysis foot baths. Gentler detoxification methods may be necessary if one is very toxic, such as a patient who has a life threatening disease, such as hepatitis or cancer.

Since clearly vast numbers of contaminants gain access to our bodies, we should encourage government and academic research institutions to study the science of detoxification. It is imperative that we need not only to prevent contamination, but also learn more about how we can help speed the removal of contaminants from the human body.

How many degenerative diseases, including heart disease, arthritis and cancer, are truly preventable given the proper technology of detoxification and education for prevention? How many dollars do we spend every year, treating these diseases? And what is the cost to society when so many of our citizens are disabled by these conditions? What price are we paying and what price will our children pay?

As long as our leaders in government and business fail to understand the holistic nature of the planet Earth, improper disbursement of toxic chemicals and electromagnetic radiation into our environment and into our bodies will continue to create diseases that result in human suffering.

As a doctor, I will continue to see women plagued by the debilitating symptoms of silicone immune disease. I will continue to see victims of Raynaud's and Morgellons disease. I will, unfortunately, continue to see and diagnose new illnesses created by the interaction of chemical, viral and biotoxins as they interact in unpredictable ways with each other and with the systems of the body. As long as corporations and governments place profit before safety and health concerns, we will continue to be plagued by a variety of mysterious diseases that are vigorously denied or ignored by the medical profession.

Indeed, we have little understanding of the long-term effects of the electromagnetic radiation from cell phones on our brains, pollution from automobile exhaust emissions on our lungs or the potential effects of pesticides, water pollution, industrial waste and nuclear power pollution on the various systems of our bodies.

In addition, we consume genetically modified food, some of which have been treated with genetically engineered microorganisms designed to consume bacteria and therefore prolong the food product's shelf life. We are beginning to see evidence that once these microorganisms are ingested, they interact within the body in unpredictable ways and may have the potential to create an entirely new class of diseases. Morgellons disease may be but one of these new diseases.[5]

Because I have treated so many women with silicone immune disease and have seen the variety of symptoms this disease can create, I am in a unique position to understand the possible consequences of new technology gone awry. In the case of faulty breast implants, chemical toxicity is at its peak because the dangerous chemicals have been introduced directly into the body. Indeed, the toxins have been surgically implanted therein.

I have had the opportunity to learn from my own

---

[5] "Staninger Interview." *Temple of Health Radio Program.* Telephone interview. 2 Aug. 2008.

experience, as well as from thousands of patients, how the body reacts to such toxicity, how the immune system functions to protect and defend the body, and how to support the body's natural capacity to detoxify itself. As my experience has grown in this emerging field, I have had the opportunity to treat patients with other types of environmental toxicity, such as Gulf War syndrome, sick building syndrome, Raynaud's disease, Morgellons disease and other toxic conditions caused or influenced by industrial pollution.

Diseases of the twenty-first century include fibromyalgia, chronic fatigue syndrome, Morgellons disease, autism, attention deficit disorder, silicone adjuvant disease, metabolic syndrome, cancer and endocrine disruption, to name just a few. Many of these emerging diseases have at their core a possible chemical or biotoxicity that is disrupting the immune and endocrine systems, as well as the neurological system in some cases. Some of these illnesses may involve genetically modified organisms gone awry. Many of the diseases are increasing in prevalence and in severity in our population, especially among children.

The majority of these diseases require holistic approaches, rather than a single treatment such as a drug. The treatment of these diseases requires an understanding of functional medicine in order to comprehend the relationships among physiological systems that are out of balance. Much can be accomplished by addressing lifestyle changes. Using supplements, herbal medicine, and other systems of nontraditional medicine can increase energy where there is evidence of energy disruption.

Our current health care system has no framework in which to place these holistic modalities. The current scientific model of medicine is geared more toward the treatment of symptoms. It is limited in its understanding of the underlying conditions that may generate the symptoms. However, in holistic medicine, we concentrate on ways we can create health, rather than on the treatment of disease. This approach designs conditions that facilitate health and wellness. In my opinion, such conditions can originate from the esoteric awareness of what the edict "as above, so below" actually means.

Twenty-first century medicine will necessarily involve a shift in our viewpoint from conventional to holistic concepts of healing. In the previous century, medical students were taught that the body is similar to a machine. When different parts of the machine break down (such as different organs, biochemical systems and physiological systems), doctors prescribe a "magic bullet" (such as an antibiotic, a pharmaceutical drug or a surgical procedure) to "fix" the problem. Physics has advanced farther than Newtonian mechanics, and with the advent of the discovery of superstring theory and quantum theory, we can no longer view the body as a machine.

Superstring theory teaches us that matter does not exist as a separate entity. All that exists are electromagnetic energy fields, which overlap and interact and are not even confined to this dimension. Therefore, we must advance our understanding of the body as the physical manifestation of these energy fields and start to study medicine not just from the viewpoint of the physical body, but endeavor to explore the different aspects of the energy body and the nature of the spiritual connections beyond the energy body.

There are, without doubt, many levels of existence outside of what we consider normal, physical reality. If we can derive a reliable means to access the higher realms of consciousness, we can achieve a broader view of our experience at this level. Seen from an elevated perspective, problems or illnesses encountered in ordinary life can serve as vehicles for spiritual growth and human evolution. Healing becomes not only about the body, but also about the emotions, mind and spirit.

The concept of higher dimensions can be understood as relating to the precessional rate of the atom. The precessional rate of the atom is that rate at which the axis of the atom completes one full precessional arc. The higher dimensions have higher vibrational rates and atoms with elevated rates of precession; therefore matter is less dense in those dimensions.

Higher dimensions exist and can be used to effect healing. According to the physicist Dr. Amit Goswami, reality consists of five "worlds of consciousness." The material dimension contains our physical reality: it is the dimension of time and space. The vital dimension contains the etheric blueprint or software of the biological body. The mental level is the domain of thoughts and reason, and it is the level on which we give meaning to our existence.

The supramental realm is where we can access the consciousness of archetypes and laws that govern creativity and manifestation. Finally, the highest dimension is the bliss dimension. The bliss realm offers us access to the unlimited ground of being with unlimited possibilities and the experience of oneness. The bliss body is the key to understanding spontaneous remission. Physical disease can be caused at all levels within the system, while healing is most powerfully enacted from the bliss dimension.[6]

In *The Quantum Doctor*, Goswami tells us that vibrational medicine operates on the principle that "downward causation" creates health. In order to choose health over disease and heal ourselves, we must transcend our ego-based perceptions and rise into the higher vibrational states of consciousness.[7] In a state of unified consciousness, for instance, when all levels are aligned with the bliss body, spontaneous healing can occur. Spiritual healings of this sort result from the "downward causation" of pure intention.

In Dr. Richard Gerber's *Vibrational Medicine* we learn that while surgeries and other allopathic techniques are effective for acute conditions such as injuries and traumas, chronic illness most often responds to vibrational techniques such as homeopathy, flower essences and other vibrationally based treatments that operate on the etheric body. The etheric body can be affected by thoughts, emotions and intentions from higher dimensions. The etheric body, in turn, will manifest these frequencies in the

---

[6] Goswami, Amit. *The Quantum Doctor: A Physicist's Guide to Health and Healing.* Charlottesvilee, VA: Hampton Roads Company, Inc., 2004. P.40
[7] Goswami: 26.

physical body.[8]

It is this multidimensional view of the world that gives meaning and purpose to what we experience in the third dimension. If the material reality is all that we experience, we live in a chaotic, fear-based world, devoid of higher meaning. We can see no purpose to our existence worthy of the suffering and pain we go through. The information we access about our current situation from the higher levels, however, not only gives meaning to our lives, but gives us hope for a better future when our current lessons are learned.

Think of the energy body as a luminous, egg-shaped energy field. This energy field not only encompasses the physical body, but also sustains it. If the field is damaged, physical decay occurs quickly. Most people cannot "see" this energy field, although clairvoyants and healers have described it for hundreds of years. Most of the information we know about the energy body is the result of the study of the chakra system. This is a system that "steps down" or transforms energy from the higher energy bodies, i.e., the spiritual, mental and emotional bodies, into the physical body. Healers often check the energy of the chakras before and after a healing session.

In the first half of the twentieth century, the author Alice Bailey wrote a series of books on spiritual teachings in philosophy, religion, science, psychology, wisdom and

---

[8] Gerber, Richard. *Vibrational Medicine: The #1 Handbook of Subtle-Energy Therapies*. Rochester, VT: Bear and Company, 2001.

healing. The material for Bailey's twenty-four books, now considered classics in esoteric literature, was conveyed to her from a nonphysical being known as Master Djwhal Khul.

Through the process of tele-thought communication, this Tibetan master of wisdom gave Bailey instructions designed to help the human species evolve through trying times. In *Esoteric Healing*, Master Djwhal Khul succinctly identifies the nature of illness when he says, "Disease is the result of inhibited soul life."[9] In other words, we enter into a state of "dis-ease" as a result of a blocked or inhibited flow of energy coming into our mental, emotional and physical bodies at the etheric level of consciousness from which we receive our life force energy. This is similar to Dr. Amit Goswami's description of "downward causation," the quantum theory principle related to health and disease.[10]

At the physical level, the body is affected by interaction with any number of material or energetic substances: food, sunlight, exercise, chemical toxins, radiation and foreign materials, i.e., dental amalgams, artificial joints, root canals, implants and suture material and electromagnetic fields (such as those from cellular and mobile phones, surrounding high tension wires and airplanes).

At the emotional level, both negative and positive emotions generated from within a person, as well as from within those to whom a person is connected, affect the energy field. Energy connections with another person need

---

[9] Bailey, Alice Anne. *Esoteric Healing*. New York: Lucis Company, 1953.
[10] Goswami: 64-66.

not necessarily be in physical proximity as is demonstrated by the example of the girl who faints when her best friend in another state dies suddenly. This is the quantum theory principle of "non-locality" described by Dr. Amit Goswami.[11] This principle is also applicable in distant healing.

At the mental level, thoughts and belief systems influence us to a degree greater than we often realize. For example, 85% of people who die from snakebites don't have enough venom in their blood streams to account for their deaths. The body's reaction to fear creates an adrenaline response, which can result in heart failure.[12]

Belief systems that regard AIDS and cancer as fatal can cause the body to shut down. Dr. Larry Dossey talks about "medical hexing" in his book, *Be Careful What You Pray For, You Might Just Get It*.[13] Dr. Dossey describes the spontaneous healing of a man with advanced cancer. The man was given an experimental drug considered by some to be a miracle cure at the time. In short order, the man's tumors disappeared. Later the man read studies suggesting that the drug was ineffective, and his cancer returned.

His doctor, acting on a hunch, gave him an injection of plain water and told him it was a new, improved version of the drug, and again the man's condition improved. Finally, the man read in the news that the American Medical

---

[11] Goswami: 66.

[12] Lewis, Howard R. and Martha E. Lewis. *Psychosomatics*. Viking P, 1975.

[13] Dossey, Larry. *Be Careful What You Pray For, You Might Just Get It*. San Francisco: Harper Collins, 1997.

Association had pronounced the drug as worthless. At that point, he completely lost faith in the drug and within a few days, he was dead.[14] One can only wonder what effects his belief system had on his immune system.

At the spiritual level, the energetic field extends beyond the energy body and beyond this dimension of time and space. Dr. Dossey calls it ERA III medicine, which involves non-local phenomena.[15] Carolyn Myss calls it "calling back your spirit."[16] You can visualize this by seeing your energy body throughout time: not only this lifetime, but also in past and perhaps even future lives.

Whenever you have a major event in your life that results in you holding a grudge or harboring hatred against an individual, a group or even a concept, you lose vital energy. Scientific studies have found that cancer patients often have endured a major life trauma within several years of the cancer being diagnosed. When we lay hands on the area of the cancer, we often "read" this information clairvoyantly.

For example, we recently treated a patient with unresectable pancreatic cancer, who had issues regarding his daughter. The situation "appeared" to me during his first healing session. When I asked him about his daughter, he replied that she had died two years prior. His wife confirmed

---

[14] Dossey: 203.

[15] Dossey, Larry. *Be Careful What You Pray For, You Might Just Get It*. San Francisco: Harper Collins, 1997.

[16] Myss, Carolyn. Anatomy of the Spirit: The Seven Stages of Power and Healing. New York: Three Rivers P, 1997.

that he was emotionally traumatized by his daughter's death. I knew that if he were willing to release this dark energy, his cancer would be more likely to regress.

Forgiveness or the release of this energy is often the key feature in the spontaneous remission of cancer. So many illnesses are related to us holding onto that which no longer serves us. We needlessly cling to old patterns of behavior, relationships that are not working and outdated patterns of thought. What causes us to hold on? It is fear: fear of loneliness, fear of separation and fear of rejection.

Healing is transmuting that fear into faith. It is important not to suppress toxic emotions, and any activity that causes the release of negativity can infuse us with energy. Besides the art of forgiveness, these practices include gratitude, praise and praying for others. Healing occurs when there is a large release of negativity rather than the suppression of such energy. The healer helps the patient to transmute that energy.

Another common feature of some cancers is that of a person who overextends herself for everyone else, but funnels little energy into her own physical body. You can visualize this by imagining that her energy body is connected to other energy bodies, such as her spouse, parents and/or children. It is even attached to other energy systems such as religions, nations, tribes and other social and political groups. If the primary direction and flow of energy is out rather than into one's energy system, disease and aging are the result. We do not age linearly; we age in spurts, usually due to stressful times in our lives.

Spiritual practices can help reverse this flow so that

energy flows into the system and health and youth result. Practices such as meditation, prayer, yoga, Tai Chi, Qi Gong, drumming, holotropic breath work, emotional release work and creative endeavors such as art and music can reverse the energy flow. Each of us also has a unique guidance system that can guide us toward health. Many call it intuition or "knowing." If we dedicate a portion of each day to checking in with this internal guidance system, we can save ourselves a lot of suffering and medical bills. The best time for this practice is probably in the morning and again prior to bed.

Checking in with ourselves for an "energy evaluation" during the day also has its benefits. Being aware of how different locations (i.e., the mall, the hospital and the workplace) affect our energy fields, how different people affect us, and how different activities and foods affect our energy level, empowers us to arrange our environment for optimal health. Becoming aware of how our thoughts and emotions affect our energy is also important. When the mind becomes still, without the interference caused by negative emotions, physical health is created.

The Role of Intuition

There is little doubt that the introduction of chemicals and biotoxins into our systems may result in physical disease if our detoxification systems are overwhelmed. Fortunately, we have our internal guidance system, which if working properly helps guide us away from exposure to harmful substances. Intuition is a sense of discernment, an inner knowing of that which will harm or help us. Intuition is not based on logic and scientific information, but is instead based on feeling and sensing. Our capacity for this type of discernment is invaluable in helping us determine which course of action is safe in spite of what popular opinion may be. A healthy sense of intuition is a major factor of spiritual protection.

Spiritual protection is created from several factors. One is the awareness of a healthy energy body so that early permutations can be detected and the responsible stimuli identified and eliminated or avoided. A healthy energy body is created from physical factors such as diet and exercise and also from spiritual practices, especially those involving quieting the mind and controlling negative thoughts.

Your awareness of your energy body will increase with spiritual practices that quiet the mind and focus on concentration. When you have developed this awareness, it is important to "tune in" to the body on a regular basis to assess the status. When you have a high enough awareness of the energy body, you can then assess multiple factors, including other people, places and even the effects of thoughts on your energy body.

Another important aspect of spiritual protection is the avoidance of negative emotional states that are produced by deceit, cheating, lying and stealing or the intent to do so. Even the thought of these can cause damage to the energy body. I know the negative energy effect of a simple "white" lie on my throat chakra or energy center. I can only imagine what the harm of intentional, repeated lying does to one's energy body. This is the mechanism for karma, the ancient law of cause and effect, which states that what you put out returns to you multiplied.

As defined in the works of Alice Bailey, "The law of karma is today a great and incontrovertible fact in the consciousness of humanity everywhere."[17] Notice that Bailey does not refer to karma as theory, but as law. As you sow, so shall you reap. As you come to understand the effects of the energy of thought or intent on the human energy field, you understand why it is important to remain "harmless." Once you seek to cause another harm, especially if you engage in deceit and lies to do so, you invite a misbalanced energy state within yourself that becomes a magnet for trouble.

Someday, the law of karma will be recognized as a physical law, especially when the energy of a thought can be measured and followed to its intended destination and back to its origin. In the meantime, remember Edgar Cayce's saying: "thoughts are things."[18]

Become aware of your thoughts and realize that they often merge with other factors to create your reality. Become aware of your feelings, as they are the sentinels for protection in this world. Learn to navigate through the day using your feelings, rather than habits, to help you with your diet, your relationships and your decisions in both your personal and professional world.

Engage frequently in spiritual practices so as to attune this guidance system to be more sensitive and give stronger

---

[17] Bailey, Alice Anne. *Esoteric Healing.* New York: Lucis Company, 1953.
[18] "Daily Thought." *Edgar Cayce Australia.* 2007. The Association for Research and Enlightenment, Inc. 25 Jan. 2009.

signals for you to recognize. Right use of will and the awareness of the "feeling" nature of your energy body constitutes your spiritual protection, so that your guardian angels do not have to work overtime.

An important part of spiritual development occurs when we realize that we not only need to recognize the protective value of intuition, but actively seek to develop our individual and collective intuition through spiritual practices. A common thread in the stories of breast implant disease survivors is that intuitive guidance, especially after periods of prayer, played a significant role in how these women were able to locate help and gain understanding of their health problems.

Many of these women had to disregard what their doctors, friends and family were telling them and look deeply within themselves to find the answers they needed. They had to discover their own intuitive guidance systems and rely on their own feelings, and finally their knowing, that their breast implants were making them ill. They had to find an internal compass to guide them in spite of all the opinions around them to the contrary.

Some patients were guided to the Internet, often in the early hours of the morning (when it may be that our guidance is strongest) where they found websites with information from other women with similar problems. They discovered not only support groups, but also clear directions toward medical professionals who could help them. They read stories of women whose conditions had improved after explantation, detoxification and further treatment of their immune systems.

As medical science keeps "looking down" to the individual cells, the genes and the molecules that make up the cell, we have to remind ourselves that we also need to "look up" and "out," into the family, into society and to our spiritual community. By focusing our attention on maintaining our spiritual, mental and emotional health, we affect the state of our physical health. Again, we see the old adage in effect: as above, so below.

An emerging popular concept is that we create our own reality. Much confusion exists if we believe that we have the power to create our reality from an ego level or the level of the separate self. If we understand that we choose, not in our ordinary state of consciousness that we call ego, but in a non-ordinary state of consciousness that is non-local or cosmic consciousness, we can learn to work as co-creators with Spirit or universal consciousness.

Essentially, in order to choose health over disease or to heal ourselves using the power of downward causation, we must transcend the ego and rise into unity consciousness. Nontraditional healing methods such as laughter, music therapy, dance therapy and art therapy are steps toward transcending the ego and moving into unity consciousness.

From a state of unified consciousness, we receive guidance, solutions are unveiled and problems are resolved. We find our intuition strengthened, the synchronicities we experience in our lives increase, and we ultimately find ourselves in a new and dynamic relationship with Spirit.

The Emerging Medical Paradigm

In allopathic medicine, there is a simple hierarchy in that

the doctor tells the patient what to do. In holistic medicine, the doctor and patient discuss problems and solutions and work together synergistically. This sometimes allows for spontaneous creativity in understanding the disease and therefore revealing the treatment. Allopathic medicine is disease control and management in a materialistic, biological view.

Holistic medicine treats more than the physical and includes emotional, mental and the spiritual remedies. Allopathic medicine works best when time is of the essence, such as in emergencies. But for chronic illnesses, holistic medicine may have an advantage. This does not mean allopathic medicine is wrong. When we shift into a paradigm of holistic and vibrational medicine, we do not reject the value of allopathic treatment. It simply opens our minds to new possibilities and expands the way we think about health and healing.

In the paradigm of holistic healing, illness can be seen as an opportunity. The Chinese ideogram for crisis is made up of symbols that represent both danger and opportunity. In disease we see the danger of suffering and death, but we also need to see an opportunity to probe more deeply into ourselves, including the supramental domain of consciousness.

Psychotherapy teaches us that conflict not properly resolved in the mental or emotional realms may become manifest on the physical plane as disease. Healing occurs when there is congruency between the mind, emotions and body. Therefore, a significant focus of holistic medicine is bringing thought, feeling and action into congruency or into harmonious vibration.

The integration of vibrational medicine into our current health care systems will be dependent on several factors, including the spiritual evolution of the practitioners and the institutions within the field of medicine. To be truly effective in the twenty-first century, medical practitioners will need to understand disease as an effect of a higher cause, a concept that involves a grasp of quantum physics as applied to health.

Our practitioners, their professional societies, hospitals and clinics, insurance companies, government regulatory agencies and policy makers must realize that the cost of health care, as well as the potential for detrimental side effects of medical treatment, can be greatly reduced by incorporating vibrational medicine into our current healthcare system.

Sadly enough, a large portion of the population may have to become ill before there is enough energy within the system to shift our institutions toward more intelligent, holistic behavior. Until then, I will continue to encourage individuals to educate themselves regarding the effects of lifestyle choices on long-term health and to develop intuitive guidance rather than blindly accepting the viewpoint of traditional medicine.

I believe that intuitive diagnosis and energy medicine, including biophysics, are the future of medicine. We will not only gain insight into the cause of injury and disease, but also more effectively treat the disturbances in the energy system using more energy-based techniques than specific medications. Preventative medicine will teach patients to become aware of their energy bodies and deal with stress before it settles into the *physical* body. As Plato said:

> *The cure of many diseases is unknown to physicians. They are ignorant of the whole which ought to be studied also. For the part can never be well unless the whole is well. This is the great error of our day in the treatment of the human body, that the physician separates the soul from the body.*[19]

Isn't it time we took Plato's words to heart and began to treat the whole patient?

---

[19] Plato, *The Dialogues of Plato*. New York: Scribner, Armstrong and Company. 1874.

Janice D.'s Story

Janice's story emphasizes the lack of support so many women find in the medical community when trying to find the source of their illness. Janice struggled with the effects of silicone implant disease for twenty years without any confirmation outside herself that she was ill. Several doctors wanted to treat her symptoms as the manifestation of psychological depression because their tests could not confirm a pre-established diagnosis. Fortunately, Janice's faith in her own sense of sanity prevailed. She knew that her condition stemmed from a physical rather than a psychological source, and she searched for answers until she found them.

Janice's story also demonstrates the long-term effects of persistent silicone toxicity. Janice's first symptoms of silicone implant disease appeared eight years after she had gotten implants (which is within the range of time the shell containing the silicone begins to break down and leak), but she struggled with a host of chronic symptoms, including extreme fatigue, aches, fevers, rashes, mental clouding, numbness and burning pain in her chest for another twenty years before her condition was correctly diagnosed. As well, the longer leaking implants remain in the body, the longer the detoxification process takes after they are removed. Janice's recovery has been slow, but her condition continues to improve.

In this story, Janice conveys a deeply spiritual message. She tells how her struggle with silicone implant disease forced her to go within herself to re-create her life to more appropriately fit the energy level she could sustain on a day-by-day basis. Her experience has resulted in some remarkable insights, and like many women on this journey, she feels it is important to share what she has learned. I consider it an honor to a part of her recovery.

"I got implants when I was twenty-five because my mother encouraged me to enlarge my breasts. She was, of course, acting out of good intentions and her desire was to help me be the best I could be. Physical beauty was a part of her world and something she valued. Besides, there was no evidence of the potential harmful consequences related to the implants at the time. I remember asking my surgeon what would happen if something went wrong with the implants. His response was simply that I would have them removed.

"I was very frightened the evening before the surgery. I stayed overnight in the hospital and couldn't sleep at all. Looking back, I think my fear was the only 'voice' I had at the time; I didn't yet have enough of my 'self' developed to acknowledge that voice. My mother's implicit message that I wasn't OK the way I was had a far-reaching impact in my life that I only came to understand many years later.

"I didn't develop symptoms or complications until eight years later. One day when I tried to pick up a large dictionary, I noticed weakness in my left hand. Over the next few weeks, I began to notice weakness up and down my left side from my face all the way down my left leg. These symptoms didn't keep me from playing racquetball or doing aerobics, but it was puzzling. I had a CAT scan to try to discover what was causing it, and no explanation was found. The weakness on my left side stayed with me over the next few years. On some days, it was more noticeable than others, but essentially, I lived a normal life. It was only many years later that I learned that neurological symptoms like left-sided weakness are a result of silicone poisoning.

"After a trip to India, I broke out in a rash. It started in my hip area and extended up toward my waist and onto my arms. Though very itchy and uncomfortable, I didn't think much of it, as travel to India brought with it all kinds of potential health hazards, from malaria to parasites to respiratory conditions related to the extreme air pollution. I had it checked when I came home and, just like with the weakness on my left side, no explanation other than 'dermatitis' was found. Many years later I learned that unexplained rashes are a symptom of silicone poisoning.

"Several years later, after months of stress related to a project at work, I suffered a severe 'burnout.' My sense of fatigue was so profound that I was flat on my back for three weeks, unable to do anything. My mind couldn't handle even reading a simple notice from work. I had no energy and it was hard to cope with doing normal activities. I had a pronounced weakness on my left side and a cool, 'Menthol' feeling above and to the left of my upper lip. At the onset of this episode, I went to the emergency room to rule out the possibility of a stroke. I had an MRI, followed by a visit to a neurologist. The doctors had no explanation for my symptoms. After three weeks, I recovered, although there was a long-term decline in my overall energy level. Again, I was puzzled, but had no explanation for what was going on.

"After this episode passed, life was fairly normal until three stressful events occurred in my life: my dad died, I lost my job, and I assisted a friend who was dying of cancer. During this time, I had an outbreak of hives. It was a tough time emotionally for me, and my energy was lagging. My doctor wanted to put me on antidepressants, but I chose not to go that way because I've always been inclined to face whatever challenges I'm having, get to the bottom of them and move on.

"I had spent many years establishing a strong sense of self and developed a sense of inner guidance that I had lacked in my earlier years. I was unwilling to allow anyone to influence me in a way that would override my hard won sense of self-appreciation and self-trust. My doctor's solution felt very wrong. The underlying message seemed to be 'You're not OK the way you are, so let's do something artificial to change you.' By this time in my life, I had enough core strength to reject that message. If I hadn't, I'm not sure I ever would have found out what was really wrong.

"I didn't feel that my doctor was my advocate or that he was interested in helping me get to the bottom of my symptoms and help me recover. I felt disregarded, lumped into that age-old category of depressed women who need to be medicated in order to cope with life. This experience compromised my trust in my doctor and left me frustrated.

"I struggled with my symptoms for the next few years, but managed to function professionally. A few days after I led a demanding five-day training, however, I completely collapsed. I lost my energy to an extreme degree, and I felt as if my life force was ebbing out of me. It was even uncomfortable for me to sit up. I was profoundly weak and had neurological symptoms including numbness that again made me wonder if I was having a stroke. Even breathing was uncomfortable. I had burning sensations in my chest area and muscle aches that produced a 'flu-ish' feeling. I couldn't sleep, was up several times at night to urinate and my hair started falling out.

"I weathered the worst of these times on my couch, propped up by pillows and wrapped up in a quilt. I thought I was dying. I went to doctors and other practitioners (an internist, a cardiologist, an acupuncturist, a nutritionist and homeopath and my chiropractor) and had many tests (MRI, extensive blood work, an EKG, echo cardiogram, carotid duplex scan, hair analysis for heavy metal toxicity, stool test for yeast, saliva test for adrenal dysfunction, tests for Lyme disease, and more), trying to discover what was wrong.

"These tests didn't reveal significant findings. Some imbalances were found, but no cause was revealed. The traditional medical doctors' evaluation was that nothing at all was wrong with me. I was unable to work except perhaps for a couple of hours a day. Going to the kitchen to make a meal took everything I had. I couldn't participate in normal life activities. My doctor continued to encourage me to take the antidepressants, but again, I said no. I felt isolated and alone; frustrated and helpless. It was very distressing to feel so ill and have no idea what was wrong.

"Over the next six months, I continued with the acupuncture treatments and the consultations with my nutritionist. I felt supported by these practitioners, but I was still in the dark. Of everyone I saw, my nutritionist was the one who started to get to the bottom of my physiological condition. We identified that my adrenals and thyroid weren't functioning properly, even though western medicine had evaluated them as normal. I began to take nutritional supplements to address these issues and made some small improvement, but still didn't know what was causing the symptoms.

"It never occurred to me that my symptoms might be related to my implants. I had a minor car accident in 2001, where the impact of the crash caused the seatbelt to bruise my chest. I went to my doctor to be checked out the next day and specifically asked if there was damage to my implants. I was told I was fine. I'm not sure if this contributed to the leakage that occurred. I also saw a plastic surgeon to remove a basal cell cancer around the same time. While there, I explained that I had implants for over twenty years and asked if he thought I needed to have them removed. His suggestion was to leave well enough alone.

"After twenty years, the mystery was finally solved when I got a surprise call from my friend, Maria, who told me she thought she knew what was making me sick. Maria had talked to a woman who had health problems due to leaking silicone implants and realized that her symptoms were remarkably similar to mine. That night, I did an Internet search and found Dr. Susan Kolb in

Atlanta, who specializes in helping women with silicone implant disease. I spoke with her by telephone the next day, and before I said much of anything, she listed a series of symptoms, all of which I had, including frequent urination at night, hair loss, neurological symptoms, burning on one side of the body (closest to the leakage) and debilitating fatigue.

"After twenty years of unexplained symptoms and wondering what was happening to me, the mystery was finally solved. I was in Atlanta to see Dr. Kolb within a couple of weeks and had my explant surgery a month later. Although my implants hadn't ruptured, I did have leakage, especially around my left breast. Over the course of the twenty-eight years I had the implants in my body, the shell had lost integrity, allowing the silicone gel to leak out.

"Dr. Kolb took out the implants, along with the scar capsule that had formed around them, and cleaned up as much of the free silicone as possible in order to give me the best chance of recovery. Dr. Kolb has developed what she calls the Silicone Immune Protocol to help the body recover from silicone implant disease. I've been taking numerous supplements in different combinations ever since my surgery four years ago to help my body deal with the silicone that remains in both my blood and tissue. The Silicone Immune Protocol addresses the ongoing challenge of my compromised energy level, as well as my accompanying neurological symptoms.

"Since swallowing pills is difficult for me (a thyroid related issue), I take many of the supplements in a shake. Doing this every day over such a long period of time is challenging. There are times I just don't want to do it anymore. As Dr. Kolb continues her research, however, there are more and more options for me. The challenge is to find the combination of protocols that work best for each individual. I continue to work with my nutritionist and Dr. Kolb to maximize my recovery.

"It's been almost two years since my explant surgery and my recovery has been a slow process. The longer the implants are in your body, the longer it takes to regain your health. Because microscopic silicone travels through the blood stream and lodges in different parts of the body, the symptoms don't just disappear when the implants are removed. Improvements are best evaluated over long periods of time, like a year, not daily, weekly or even monthly. I can sustain more activity now, but my condition still compromises the quality of how I feel and what I'm able to each day.

"I still struggle with low life force, flu-like feelings, burning sensations in my body and difficulty sleeping. There are moments, perhaps hours or even a few days, when I feel better, even 'well.' In periods like these, I think that perhaps one day this will be over. But so far, inevitably, I pay a price for those days when I exert a lot of energy because I've chosen to do something I love or be with people I love.

"Usually the good days are followed by some extremely bad days, and those days I feel just about as bad as I felt in the early days. That's the scary part. It's hard to explain it to your friends who often offer what they intend as supportive comments like 'We're all more tired these days' or 'We're just getting older.' I realize these people are well meaning, but I'm left with a feeling that they can never understand what I'm dealing with.

"The good days are more frequent now and that gives me hope. I have found that the only way to cope with these bad times is to stay in the present (the most profound life lesson in any setting) and be appreciative of what I can do, not what I can't do. I am able to work more of a full time schedule now, but I still have to be careful about my activity level. I sometimes have bad lupus-like episodes where all I can do is lie down. I am a life and business coach and have been lucky to have a way of making a living that allows me to work out of my home. With my condition as it is, I would be unable to sustain a normal job.

"When I told my doctor that I had discovered what was wrong and was going to have the surgery, he cautioned me against it, saying that some people get worse after the surgery. Although there is some truth to that (due to the possibility of silicone spillage during explantation, which can cause a worsening of symptoms) it was crystal clear to me that I couldn't walk around with poison slowly leaking more and more into my body.

"I'm very happy I found out what was wrong, and I would like other women who might be suffering from the same thing to know there is help. My experience with my own doctor was very poor. His focus was on giving me medications to manage what he saw as depression. While it wasn't an easy time emotionally, there was much more to the picture than my emotional condition. I felt discounted by my doctor. He didn't go far enough as my advocate in terms of figuring this out. When I presented him with valid new information, he doubted that silicone leakage could be the cause of my illness and showed no interest in reading the research Dr. Kolb had provided. I found that in the medical community, doctors disbelieve the existence of this 'silicone' disease, caused by leaking implants. They disbelieve it because studies haven't been done correctly to prove it. By taking refuge in the lack of 'scientific proof,' they discount the very real suffering of thousands of women.

"I have recently found that I need another surgery to remove a lymph node that has silicone trapped in it under my left arm. Dr. Kolb tells me this isn't unusual for women in my condition. If the silicone stays there, there is a chance for more symptoms. Again, other doctors I consulted discouraged me from this surgery with comments ranging from 'It's nothing to be concerned about' to 'You've gained a few pounds; maybe it's just fat.'

"It was aggravating to experience such a wholesale lack of interest and belief within the medical community. I found complete support and understanding, however, from Dr. Kolb and trusted her knowledge, expertise, integrity and support. She personally returned my telephone call within hours of leaving her that first message, and from that moment I have trusted the entirety of my experience with her. She understood, and in my condition, that meant everything to me.

"I trust that Dr. Kolb has the depth of knowledge to lead me to my best possible recovery. She is an inspiration in this little researched disease. She's been an angel in my life. Looking back, finding Dr. Kolb was like finding a needle in a haystack. After being so ill and in the dark for so long, finding her so instantly when I finally had an inkling of what might be wrong seemed like a miracle. She seemed heaven sent. She was second in an internet search that revealed thousands of possibilities related to leaking silicone implants. It was an incredible relief to get good information from someone who clearly had the right expertise and offered help and hope.

"Every step of the way from there on seemed guided. The flight to Atlanta from California was difficult to make as I was very weak. I arrived at night and had an appointment with Dr. Kolb the next day. When I arrived at her office I was frightened and in bad shape from the trip. I was shown to her office and when I walked in, I saw a very large and beautiful statue of an angel. I felt without a doubt that I had been guided to the right place.

"Dr. Kolb has so many gifts and among them is her gift for hands-on healing. As we ended the medical part of the appointment, she explained that she understood how rough the travel is when you feel so ill. She knew this because she had experienced it herself. She said, 'You feel like you're going to die, but you don't.' That just about summed up my experience of the last six months. Then she offered to do a hands-on healing treatment. It brought me great peace and assurance that I was in good hands. Since then Dr. Kolb has remained accessible and a cutting edge advocate for the thousands of women who are coping with silicone disease.

"I have been significantly changed by my illness. It helped me take the final step to a lifelong search for wholeness, finding that I am the source of the answers I seek (versus seeking the answers outside of myself). I have learned how to focus on what I want instead of what I don't want. I have learned how to appreciate myself and the 'offerings' that appear in my life based on that pinpointed focus. I have learned that I have a choice of where I put my focus and that my thoughts create my emotions, which in turn set my vibration, attracting more of whatever matches that vibration.

"I have learned that to attract more of what I want; I must be at peace with what is. Knowing what I want and focusing on it, feeling the joy of it as if it were already here is the key to attracting that very thing. As I experience this, increasingly more and more miracles appear in my life."

-8-
LESSONS

"Trials are but lessons that you failed to learn,
presented once again."
Anonymous

There are many different levels from which we can look at
the spiritual meaning of disease. Take the example of a
capsular contracture around a breast implant. On the
physical level, this is a tightening of the scar tissue around
an implant causing firmness, sometimes discomfort and
upward migration of the implant. Capsular contracture is
thought to be secondary to subclinical bacterial
contamination around the implant, which causes a
shortening of the scar capsule. It is more common when the
implant is placed in the submammary rather than a submuscular location, probably because of the disruption of
breast ducts containing small amounts of bacteria. When the
implant is placed below the muscle, there is less contact with
bacteria and consequently less chance of infection. Could
there be other aspects to the development of a capsular

contracture other than this subclinical infection?

In 1991, a young woman asked me to perform a breast augmentation procedure through the axillary approach in order to avoid scars on the breast. I generally recommend a submammary approach because there are usually fewer complications than with the axillary approach. The incision made in this approach is underneath the breast just above the fold where the breast begins, and the scar is hardly even visible. In meditation prior to the surgery, I was shown that this patient would develop a right-sided capsular contracture after the surgery.

At this point while still in the meditation, I asked if I should perform the operation in view of the advanced knowledge of the complication. The answer I received was that I should proceed with the surgery because the patient needed to learn to detach from the physical. The following day, the operation was carried out with no problems and my patient did well for a week. Then her uncle pulled her arm with some force, which led to swelling on the right side. A short while later, this developed into a mild but noticeable capsular contracture.

The patient was not happy with the breast asymmetry caused by the contracture and asked if I could fix the problem. This was in the days before the endoscope was widely used to correct capsular contracture, so I told her that I could correct the problem, but that the procedure would leave a scar on the lower part of the breast. This left her with a dilemma. She had the choice of living with a capsular contracture or having a scar on her breast in an area she felt would be visible. Either way, she would necessarily have to learn a lesson in detachment. This experience would ultimately teach her to detach her identity from her physical body and identify more strongly with her spiritual being.

After witnessing this occurrence, I realized that we're often put in such situations when it is time for us to learn our spiritual lessons. In times like these, we will learn the lessons we need for spiritual advancement, no matter what choice we make. Some lessons may be predestined to be successful, but only after we've gone through them can we understand how significant the changes they created within us are. Indeed, they often affect us at the deepest level of our being.

We can analyze the spiritual lessons associated with the breast implant dilemma from a number of perspectives. Because breast implant disease does not occur naturally, we must examine its implications as human-created disease and a sociological occurrence. What breakdown in the spiritual systems of our society resulted in the manifestation of this disease and the controversy surrounding it? How can we heal and protect ourselves from this kind of mis-creation?

The choice to undergo breast augmentation is an individual decision, but only if the choice is made freely and with the benefit of accurate information. A woman's choice is necessarily influenced by the culture in which she lives and the culture bears some responsibility for her decision. She must place her trust not only in her doctor and the medical community, but also in the corporations who manufacture the implants and the government charged with assessing their safety and effectiveness. Finally, she must subscribe to a societal view of beauty to which she wishes to conform.

Lessons Learned from Patients

Historically, when scientists have wanted to learn about a new disease, they have studied the patients who have the disease. However, if the intent is to avoid studying the disease or to prove the disease does not exist, "scientific" research can be misused to "prove" that, as well. Indeed, scientists who know enough about the phenomena they are studying have the ability to determine the variables that will be used in the study. They can either consciously (or even unconsciously) manipulate data to produce an outcome they desire. The peer-reviewed research that was most helpful in determining the course of this clinical illness consisted of studies on women who were ill.

It is not possible to perform epidemiological studies on diseases that have not yet been characterized, because such studies seek to classify symptoms into disease categories that have already been established. The epidemiological studies that were so widely quoted in the press and by the plastic surgeons serve only to show that silicone causes a disease different from the classical autoimmune illnesses currently known.

What makes breast implant disease so interesting is that it is an iatrogenic disease or an illness caused by the medical profession. From a spiritual perspective, it was likely one of the most important tests given to the medical profession in the last century. It is most interesting that during the last wave of the controversy, the majority of plastic surgeons, rheumatologists and neurologists were of the opinion that silicone gel implants did not cause systemic disease. This is probably because the organizations representing these groups issued public statements to that effect, supposedly after a review of the pertinent peer-reviewed literature.

These physicians, no doubt, trusted the information they were given by their professional organizations. There were, however, a few more observant individual doctors who looked at their patients and realized they were ill with a disease that was not yet known to medical science. In consulting with these rare individuals about mutual patients, I have noticed several qualities they share.

First, they are more intelligent than the average physician in that they think independently and have better observation skills. Second, they do their own investigative research. They read the medical literature and search alternative avenues for answers to their patient's problems. Sometimes they are related to a very sick patient and recognize the temporal relationship of the systemic illness to the onset of chest wall symptoms many years after implantation. The common quality that these doctors share is that they know that they do not know everything about medicine and are willing to learn from their patients.

My patient population had clinical signs and symptoms that mirrored what was going on in my own body as a result of breast implants. I listened carefully to their stories and the course of events in their life, for I was determined to find out what was causing this disease and how to treat it. I had at my disposal the ability to interview anyone who knew more than I did about any aspect of this problem either on my radio or television program. This was a great benefit, for I found out early that many doctors who were closed-lipped about their treatments of these patients were more than happy to talk freely of their treatments and theories on the air.

It was from these interviews that I learned that the most effective treatments were holistic detoxification programs. I also learned that programs designed to support the immune system were highly effective, as bacterial, viral and fungal infections appear to run rampant in this patient population. Of course, I had myself on which to experiment, as my doctors so kindly left a sufficient amount of silicone in my chest wall. Consequently, I was very motivated to pursue detoxification programs and holistic methods to support my own immune system. This led me on a search through holistic medicine and the evidence-based approach to solving difficult problems.

The standard medical approach emphasizes the use of the random, double-blind, controlled clinical study to prove or disprove the effectiveness of a given therapy. The double-blind study is supposed to cancel out the effect called "the placebo effect." The placebo effect is a mind-body connection through which up to thirty percent of patients may experience a positive treatment outcome simply because they believe the therapy will be effective.

One of my favorite parodies of the double-blind study

method was reported in *The British Medical Journal.* The satirical study showed that the effect of wearing a parachute while jumping out of a plane led to a positive outcome.[1] The point of the article is that we don't have to conduct this experiment with an equal number of patients jumping out of airplanes, half of which have parachutes and half which do not have parachutes, in order to deduce the outcome.

We already know that the patients jumping out of airplanes without parachutes would most likely not survive. We can rely on the evidence that patients safely jump out of airplanes with functioning parachutes as evidence that parachutes are effective. This would be evidence-based medicine. No matter how many "scientific" studies are published indicating that no link can be established between breast implants and autoimmune symptoms in the patient population, I have seen the evidence of it in my patients and have experienced it in my own body. The best source of information in diagnosing and treating an illness is the patients themselves.

It is obvious that the current studies for breast implant pre-market approvals for the FDA are completely inadequate given the time frames and the range of toxicities that may be involved in the pathophysiology of breast implant disease. It would, no doubt, be much more valuable to study those women who have developed systemic illness

---

[1] Smith, Gordon C. and Jill P. Pell. "Hazardous Journey: Parachute Use to Prevent Death and Major Trauma Related to Gravitational Challenge: Systematic Review of Randomised Controlled Trials." *British Medical Journal* 327 (2003): 1459-461.

from their breast implants, rather then to perform studies on women who have yet to become ill. One is much more likely to be able to characterize a new disease if they actually study those patients who are ill, rather than study a group of patients who are not.

It would also lend more credibility to the research if the principal investigators in these studies were not plastic surgeons with a vested interest in the studies' outcomes. It can hardly be considered ethical (or rational) for surgeons whose livelihoods are derived from breast implant surgeries to conduct unbiased scientific research. The public and, indeed, many physicians, unaware of these conflicts of interest, easily accept the studies' findings, naively believing that there is a lack of evidence supporting the development of systemic disease in breast implant patients.

What the general public, as well as many physicians, don't realize is that the women who participated in the research used to gain FDA approval had their implants less than five years.[2,3,4] Yet it is evident in the scientific literature on breast implants that the shell containing the silicone loses integrity between eight and fourteen years after

---

[2] US FDA/CDRH. "Breast Implant Questions and Answers (2006)." *U S Food and Drug Administration.* 2006. 10 Feb. 2009.
http://www.fda.gov/cdrh/breastimplants/qa2006.html#s2
[3] "Breast Implant Clinical Studies." *Love Your Look.* 2007. Mentor Corporation. 19 Jan. 2009.
http://www.loveyourlook.com/Breast-Implants/clinical-studies.aspx
[4] "Frequently Asked Questions about MemoryGel Implants." *Mentor.* 2007. Mentor Corporation. 19 Jan. 2009
http://www.memorygel.com/FAQs.aspx

implantation, allowing silicone gel to leak into the chest cavity.[5,6,7] Symptoms caused by silicone and chemicals leaching into the body are not likely to appear in women who have had their implants for less than five years, making the FDA approval studies virtually worthless.

So what is the broader lesson in all of this? First it is important to understand that governmental agencies do not necessarily have as their first priority the protection of public health. Far too often the interests of corporate entities weigh more heavily than do the interests of the public. The system is set up to allow manipulation of the FDA's approval process, often through scientific research controlled by special interest groups.

It only becomes obvious later on, after FDA approval has been granted, that there may have been serious flaws in the studies reviewed by the FDA. By then, however, the damage to the public may have already been done, and the flurry of class-action lawsuits spring up along with the FDA recall of the medication or device. It would be a better idea to have an independent review process made up of a panel of members who are not financially invested in the drug or

---

[5,] Robinson, O. Gordon, Edwin L. Bradley, and Donna S. Wilson. "Analysis of Explanted Silicone Implants: A Report of 300 Patients." *Annals of Plastic Surgery* 34 (1995): 1-6.

[6,] Cohen, Benjamin E., Thomas M. Biggs, Ernest D. Cronin, and Donald R. Collins. "Assessment and Longevity of the Silicone Gel Breast Implant." *Plastic and Reconstructive Surgery Journal* 99 (1997): 1697-601.

[7] Pfleiderer, B., T. Campbell, C. A. Hulka et al. "Silicone Gel-Filled Breast Implants in Women: Findings at H-1 MR Spectroscopy." *Radiology* 201 (1996): 777-83.

device. These impartial parties would be free to raise appropriate questions and concerns during the approval process, which could then be addressed prior to the release of the drug or device.

A case in point is the example of the potentially harmful effects of cell phone radiation. An article in the Winter 2002 edition of *Anti-Aging Medical News* reviews the scientific data of studies performed by Dr. George Carlo and other researchers.[8] The evidence presented by Dr. Carlo shows that frequent use of cellular telephones is associated with increased permeability of the blood brain barrier, increased risk of genetic damage within cells and adverse cellular effects due to thermal stress.

All of these conditions may predispose individuals who frequently use the cellular telephones (especially close to the head) to have an increased risk of neuroepithelial malignancies (malignant brain tumors), as well as an increased risk of acoustic neuromas (benign tumors of the VIII (eighth) cranial nerve which controls hearing and balance). The cell phone industry hired Dr. Carlo to perform research to show that cell phones did not pose a public health risk.

According to his book, *Cell Phones: Invisible Hazards in the Wireless Age*, when his research failed to prove that cell

---

[8] Goldman, Robert and Rondal Klatz. "Cellular Phone Radiation and Potential Risks to the Human Brain." *Anti-Aging Medical News*. Winter, 2002. 26 Jan. 2009.
http://www.worldhealth.net/assets/publications/AAMN_Winter02scr.pdf.

phone radiation was safe for human use, he was forced to find other routes to inform the public of his scientific findings.[9] This is but another example of the crisis of ethics in corporate entities that are financially invested in the research they fund. We hear increasingly often about companies who manipulate research findings and misuse their influence to garner public favor in an effort to sell more of their product.

In many cases, by the time studies are even performed, the product may already be in widespread use, endangering unwitting consumers. Those scientists and other individuals who may have knowledge of the risks are often actively suppressed or ridiculed or forced underground by the corporations in question.

The danger of cell phone use is similar to that of silicone implants in that the mechanism of injury may be multi-factorial, meaning that more than one system within the human body may be affected. Because the span of time needed for a serious adverse outcome to develop (such as a brain tumor in the case of cellular telephone radiation or an increased risk of lung, colon or brain cancer in the case of silicone breast implant patients) is often ten to fifteen years, it is easy to develop studies which will fail to show these adverse associations.

Any scientific researcher who understands how variables

---

[9] Carlo, George and Martin Schram. Cell Phones: Invisible Hazards in the Wireless Age: An Insider's Alarming Discoveries about Cancer and Genetic Damage. New York: Carroll & Graf Publishers. 2001.

in a given study will affect each other can skew an outcome. Since the scientists designing the study can control these variables, the outcome can be assured if that is their intent. The public unfortunately is unaware that the experiment's design can specifically be used to produce the desired result. The public has too often accepted the premise that the scientific method is flawless and beyond reproach. They have bought into the idea that science is somehow infallible.

Even when the intent of a study is honorable, scientists who have a vested interest in the outcome of a given study may not be able to remain objective and unbiased. When corporations fund the research on new products they produce, can we trust the results to be "scientific"? This conflict of interest sets up a scenario in which the very basis of science, objective observation, is compromised.

Oversight of the FDA approval process, as well as the design and execution of the scientific studies, should not be in the hands of corporations or physicians with a vested interest in the outcome of this research. Research into product safety should be handled by an independent research facility, which is neither controlled by the government nor by the corporations who have developed the products or devices.

The cost of such research could be funded by a joint funding program involving monies from more than one source so that no one entity controls the funding. Therefore, excessive influence by one interested party may be avoided.

During a recent radio broadcast, I interviewed Colette Baron-Reid, a clairvoyant, regarding her book *Remembering the Future*.[10] When I mentioned that silicone breast implants were being released again for general use, she predicted that there would be another class-action lawsuit due to the fact that these implants would react adversely with something in the food supply.

As I had just reviewed the scientific paper given by Dr. Hildegarde Staninger on her findings of silicone, silica and high-density polyethylene in Morgellons patients,[11] I realized that Colette's prediction was inevitable. I was also seeing patients with Morgellons Disease who had eaten significant quantities of luncheon meat (which had likely been treated with a nanotech coating of high-density polyethylene around a viral phage) develop exacerbations of their symptoms. I realized, as well, that information is readily available from high levels, which this clairvoyant easily accessed, and I recognized that it foolish for us not to use such information.

If we could devise or evolve a way to access accurate information from the higher dimensions, we could not only use it in the treatment of diseases, but in their prevention. Information could be gathered from different clairvoyant sources that could then be cross-referenced with each other

---

[10] Baron-Reid, Colette. *Remembering the Future: The Path to Recovering Intuition.* CA, Carlsbad: Hay House, Inc. 2006.

[11] Staninger, Hildegarde. *Fiber Made of High Density Polyethylene (HDPE).* Laboratory report. Lakewood, CA: Integrative Health International, LLC, 2006.

to determine areas of concern. The direction given by the clairvoyant information would allow the scientific studies to be designed in the most efficient manner. Potential problems with a new drug or device could be identified early in the process, and the high cost of potentially deadly side effects, not to mention costly litigation, could be avoided.

Lessons for the Patients

Developing a debilitating disease whose cause is unknown to the medical community may be viewed as an extraordinarily arduous spiritual path. Yet in spite of extreme challenges, patients who develop immune dysfunctions as a result of their breast implants are often able to navigate through the misinformation and the lack of support from medical community to find healing. Ultimately, they find that they heal, not only on the physical level, but on the emotional, mental and spiritual levels as well.

Because the medical condition caused by breast implants is at its very core an iatrogenic disease (meaning that it is brought on by doctors or the medical profession), and the patients have received so little support from the medical community, they are frequently angry and disillusioned with the health care system. Yet because they are often very ill, they are still dependent on health care system.

I have observed that patients fare much better if they are able to release this anger or at least channel it into more constructive outlets. I encourage the patients to seek out holistically minded physicians and other healthcare practitioners who have open minds.

I refer them to the website of the American Holistic Medical Association (http://www.holisticmedicine.org) for a list of holistic physicians in their area.

Pamela Jones, MD, is a prime example of someone who found the capacity to channel the devastating emotions created by this disease into productive work. Using her experience as a medical doctor and a psychiatrist, she produced a remarkable website on Human Adjuvant Disease. (http://www.freewebs.com/implants). Her website contains up-to-date information for patients as well as doctors. She also offers emotional support to other women struggling with this disease and works tirelessly on their behalf to connect them with appropriate medical care.

While many doctors remain in a state of denial about breast implant disease, I often find physicians who are more than willing to learn about this disease after they see the remarkable improvements in their patient's health after explantation and detoxification procedures. I have received phone calls from neurologists, endocrinologists and pulmonary medicine doctors inquiring as to how my treatment program could affect their patient's neurological system, endocrine system and pulmonary function to such a great degree.

One lesson learned in retrospect from the patients' standpoint is to take responsibility for their own treatment. Many patients regret that they did not gather information about surgical procedures from sources other than just their plastic surgeon before getting implants. Patient after patient tells me that their plastic surgeons did not tell them about the possibility of systemic complications.

Many women who have breast implant surgery have no idea that the possibility of an autoimmune disorder even exists. While plastic surgeons may not inform their patients of the toxic potential of breast implants, information about such complications can be found on the Internet. However, the patient herself must take the responsibility to be informed and not trust blindly in medical authority. True informed consent can only be achieved through a process of due diligence in which the patient does her own research.

Another advantage of a patient doing her own research is that if a complication should arise, the patient is informed in advance and can respond to seek appropriate treatment quickly. Unfortunately, there is no guarantee that the patient's plastic surgeon will be familiar with that particular problem or how to treat it.

The patient is in a much better position to find the help she needs if she makes herself familiar with the complication she is experiencing than if she merely depends on the advice of her doctor. I find it interesting that so many plastic surgeons have told their patients that saline implants are safe and that if their implants should leak, the saline will be reabsorbed into the body without any problems.

These plastic surgeons should be familiar with the professional literature, which indicates that bacteria and mold can grow inside saline breast implants. Infection around a foreign body is a well-known complication in medicine, and saline breast implants, especially textured implants with their increased propensity to harbor microorganisms, are no exception. Chronic pain around an implant signals an infection. It is rare to see a full-blown infection with redness and fever around a breast implant, and if this is present, there is usually an infected seroma or serum collection around the device. Often the pain will radiate into the axilla or armpit, as this is the path of the lymphatic drainage. I have had many patients come to me whose doctors have failed to diagnose such an infection.

Another lesson women often learn through their dilemmas with breast implant disease is to find a physician who will listen and learn. This condition is largely unknown and little understood in the medical community and research into its effective treatment is a continuing process. Women often encounter doctors who know nothing about it, and ironically, some of these doctors may treat these patients with a condescending attitude.

Many women faced with this illness encounter doctors who minimized the seriousness of their symptoms and treat them as if they are hypochondriacs or hysterics. Doctors often prescribe antidepressants to these women, believing the symptoms of this devastating physical illness exist only their minds. This attitude is an indication of ignorance, not superiority, and a woman who confronts such an attitude has to remain true to herself and trust in her own sense of inner knowing.

Women who see this kind of behavior in their doctors must realize that there is very little chance they can be of any real help. They should first take steps to protect themselves from such unhealthy projections, and immediately begin to seek the help of another, more qualified doctor.

Indeed, if a patient's condition does not improve under

the guidance of a health care provider for any reason, it is imperative for her to seek help from alternative physicians. There can be any number of reasons particular physicians may or may not be effective with particular patients or classes of patients. It is important for women who suffer from breast implant complications to find a healer who is a match for them.

Because illness associated with breast implants can be systemic as well as localized, it is important to find a plastic surgeon who understands the disease. Many women, who have been treated with partial rather than total capsulectomies (removal of the scar capsule around the implant), find themselves in a far worse condition than if they had not had the explantation surgery.

If the surgeon is not familiar with the importance of performing the procedure "en bloc" (removing the implant and scar capsule in one piece with the silicone contained within), the silicone gel can spill outside the capsule and into the chest wall. Women who have had gross spillage of the silicone gel outside the capsule may find themselves quite ill from chemical toxicity.

I know how sick one can become in such a case from personal experience. My scar capsules were not removed at the time of my explant surgery because the scar tissue surrounding them had adhered to my ribcage. For several months after my surgery, I found myself seriously ill.

It is also important to find doctors who can recommend treatment programs for detoxification of the chemical and biotoxins, as well as treatment of the neurological, immune and endocrine problems. The best outcomes occur when the surgeon understands and treats the concurrent bacterial, fungal and viral infections frequently found in these patients due to the immune deficiency. Specific immune therapies prior to and during surgery and in the postoperative period are also important to avoid postoperative exacerbations of infections. As silicone and saline breast implant disease affects so many of the body's systems, a holistic approach to the treatment of these patients is necessary.

Surgeons who do not believe that breast implants cause systemic disease are not able to effectively treat women who are sick from their breast implants. An understanding of how the toxicity resulting from breast implants affects the bodies systems is essential because certain medical treatments must be rendered concurrently with the surgical treatment.

Many patients have had to undergo secondary surgeries because total capsulectomies were not performed or surgical drains were not in place for a sufficient length of time and recurrent seromas developed and became infected. Many surgeons do not recognize the importance of removing enlarged silicone filled lymph nodes as part of the primary procedure, especially with ruptured silicone gel implants. Consequently, patients have to return for additional procedures, which could have been performed at the time of the explantation.

Management of immune and endocrine problems is critical in the perioperative period of silicone patients, for if not properly managed, the patients can have prolonged infections from surgery, as well as endocrine complications, such as significant adrenal insufficiency.

Apart from lessons applicable to understanding one's illness and how to best seek treatment to remedy it, there are several deeper core issue spiritual lessons for women with breast implant disease. A very common spiritual lesson is to learn to love yourself despite your perceived imperfections, especially as relates to your body. If you are seeking to find love outside yourself in order to fill an emptiness created by lack of love for yourself, this strategy will necessarily fail. Some women were encouraged to enlarge their breasts by their boyfriends or husbands to be more sexually attractive to their partners.

Some women felt that with breast enlargement they would be more attractive to others and thus gain their love. Some women sought to save a relationship by enlarging their breasts. Many women with very little breast development or with asymmetrical breasts saw breast augmentation is a way to correct a congenital deformity. Many women underwent breast reconstruction using tissue expanders and or breast implants as a way to correct an acquired deformity after cancer surgery.

As a plastic surgeon trained in both cosmetic and reconstructive surgery, I do not have a problem helping patients achieve a more normal physical state, especially if they have a congenital or acquired deformity. I feel I had an acquired deformity myself and understand the benefits of breast augmentation for those who have little to no breast tissue. I also understand that I am not my breasts or my body. I am not my emotions or even my thoughts.

My consciousness is not limited to my physical body or even limited in time or space. If I harbor limiting thoughts in my consciousness, such as the belief that my self worth is related to my breast size (or in any way related to the appearance of my body), then I will live in a reality that these limiting thoughts create and attract relationships that support my belief systems. It is much more fulfilling to live in a world in which these limiting thoughts do not create your reality, and the relationships that you attract are not dependent on your physical appearance.

Since physical beauty fades with time, you may find yourself uncomfortable with what you see in the mirror. If you believe that others only love to for your physical beauty, these thoughts create a destiny that might be very lonely.

Chronic illness, especially when iatrogenic (created by the medical profession), can give rise to negative emotions, which make healing even more difficult. Many women sought out others in support groups on the Internet for help and advice with the problems this disease creates.

Some of the negative emotions expressed by my patients and the women in the support groups concern feelings of worthiness or lack of self-love, guilt, and anger. Women struggle with the limiting belief that their worthiness is related to their physical bodies, not only in their families but also in society. The breasts are central to a women's sense of femininity and when their breasts do not develop or are taken away by disease and surgery, feelings of inadequacy can result.

Many women carrying the heavy burden of guilt that they have ruined their lives and reneged on their responsibilities to their families because of a decision to enlarge their breasts with an implant that they were told by their doctors was safe and would last a lifetime. They feel guilty that they did not do more research and trusted the word of their physician. They feel guilty that they have not been there for their children or their families. They feel guilty because their husbands have left them. They feel guilty because they are too sick to hold down a job or take care the house and too mentally confused to figure a way out of their dilemma.

Doctors tell them their illness is not related to their breast implants, but in their hearts they know this is not true. This disease is truly a significant spiritual test of one's intuition and ability to manifest that which one needs.

When a woman becomes chronically ill, a busy schedule of activities can come to a grinding halt. Because she is too ill to embark on other pursuits, she now has the time for spiritual development. In early 2005, I developed a serious case of viral pneumonia, which had me bedridden for five weeks. I could do very little other than rest and listen to my inner guidance.

Through a series of dreams and meditations, I received instructions on how to survive. I was guided as to which supplements and treatments, such as acupuncture and massage, would help my condition. I was also specifically guided not to go to the hospital for traditional medicine has little to offer in the treatment of viral pneumonia. I believe my patients are often similarly guided to figure out a way out of their health dilemmas.

Many of my patients come to me by referral from other patients, and many come to me by way of the Internet, as it has not been particularly safe for me to appear publicly in the media and speak about these issues. Oddly enough, the return of silicone to the market along with the Dow Corning lawsuit settlement, has allowed me to speak more freely as the vested interests of the doctors and implant companies are no longer threatened.

I believe that there comes a time in one's spiritual development when one is faced with a grave crisis, often life-threatening, and the solution to this problem lies solely in following one's intuitive guidance. Indeed, if one heeds the advice of outside advisors, serious problems arise. It may be that during these times, techniques such as prayer, meditation, dream analysis and listening to the still, small voice within are the only way out, other than death.

Silicone illness may have a significant mortality rate due to complications from systemic infections from an impaired immune system. One of the nurses informed me that half of her patient list had died in the twelve years it took Dow Corning to begin making payments to women from the settlement.

I believe that with proper treatment, including surgery to remove the silicone implants, scar capsule and involved lymph nodes, treatment of the immune system, treatment of the concurrent infections, and detoxification of the chemicals and biotoxins left in the body, we can certainly prevent these patients from dying prematurely and give them hope for relief from a painful and progressive systemic illness.

After following many of the Internet support groups for many years, I am happy to report that the negative emotions are now less intense and less common than they were in earlier years, and the positive emotions and support that the women provide each other are more prevalent. It may be that the anger and frustration with the medical profession and implant companies has burned itself out and has been replaced with a sense of disbelief that government agencies such as the FDA, the medical establishment and the corporations responsible for this fiasco have learned nothing from it. As Karl Marx is often paraphrased as saying, "History repeats itself, first as tragedy, second as farce."

Lessons for the Medical Profession

There are many potential lessons inherent in this catastrophe for the medical profession. My hope is that in the future the profession might evolve to incorporate the following tenets of wisdom:

1. Listen to the patient and he or she will tell you the diagnosis.

2. Use similarities in clinical history timelines from many patients to figure out the disease and its cause.

3. Do not trust the newspaper and media headlines. Public relation companies working for the corporations often influence them. Realize that our media has not been a free press for some time and that it is heavily influenced by corporate and government biases.

4. Read the medical literature, including papers not specifically in your area of specialization.

5. Understand that epidemiology studies are of no use in the study of new diseases, at least until the diseases have been defined and/or categorized.

6. Look for similar clinical pictures and other settings

to understand causation.

7. Ascertain the cause of the problem or disease, and treat the cause rather than simply treating the symptoms.

8. Maintain a sense of compassion and learn to recognize patients who are truly ill. Do not dismiss a patient's illness simply because you do not understand its cause.

9. Understand that breast implant disease is an iatrogenic disease and that all of us in the medical profession have a special obligation to seek out and find treatment for this condition, especially because it is iatrogenic. Failure to do so results in specific karmic consequences.

Lessons for Corporate Manufacturers

There are also lessons to be learned for the corporations who produce and market breast implants. Again, I believe these lessons remain unlearned, but there is potential for them to be learned in the future. Despite paying out billions of dollars to injured consumers, little evidence suggests that the corporations promoting breast implants have gained wisdom through their experience in this controversy. In the future, I hope the corporations involved realize the importance of the following lessons:

1. Understand that with any new technology there is a likelihood of problems arising after the initial product development and testing phase, which could not have been recognized during the research phase. Long-term

implications of new technology on the human body cannot be ascertained by short-term studies. Setting up systems to identify these problems as quickly as possible after they arise, before significant widespread damage has occurred may prevent class-action lawsuits.

2. Public opinion cannot be permanently manipulated by public relations strategies. Such manipulations are temporary and historically have been exposed by whistleblowers. After exposure, there is a public outcry that the corporation has been deliberately dishonest. The public can be very forgiving, but only if they feel the corporation has been honest and tried to correct their problems rather than covering them up.

3. Early recognition and correction of a potentially damaging problem is good business. You can outmaneuver your competition by making the public aware of your vigilance and acceptance of responsibility for the problem.

4. Companies that consistently violate ethical principles in business are no longer in business, so the creation of a strong ethical foundation within corporations is a good survival strategy. Dow Corning, for instance, was forced into bankruptcy proceedings after thousands of lawsuits were filed against them for hiding research that indicated silicone was not safe.[12]

---

[12] "Frontline: Breast Implants on Trial: Breast Implant Chronology." *PBS*. 1995-2008. 19 Jan. 2009
http://www.pbs.org/wgbh/pages/frontline/implants/cron.html

Lessons for the Government

There are also lessons for our government. Although from a government standpoint, we don't seemed to have learned much, I still hope the following lessons will be learned in the future:

1. The current system of drug and device approval needs to be redesigned because it is simply not working. The problems inherent in its systemic structure need to be carefully analyzed and addressed. As it stands now, political and corporate interests are consistently placed ahead of public health concerns. We need to be able to trust our government officials to make clear, unbiased decisions that are in the best interest of our national health.

2. The "precautionary principle" necessarily needs to be incorporated into our regulatory agencies.[13] The precautionary principle is a moral and political precept, which states that if it is within our power, we have an ethical imperative to prevent rather than merely to treat disease, especially in the face of scientific uncertainty. This principle goes so far as to state that in the absence of scientific consensus, the burden of proof falls on the shoulders of those advocating an action or, in this case, a product. The precautionary principle can be seen as an

---

[13] Raffensperger, Carolyn, "Precautionary Principle: Bearing Witness to and Alleviating Suffering, Part 1." *Environmental Research Foundation.* 22 Jan. 2003. 26 Jan 20
http://www.rachel.org/en/node/5625

extension of the ancient medical principle of "First, do no harm" to social, business and government institutions.

3. The FDA and other regulatory agencies need to develop and pay careful attention to "early warning systems." Systems need to be implemented to signal problems with new and evolving devices and/or drugs. Increased attention to MedWatch forms, for example, could indicate clusters of problems around certain new products. (My office recently called the FDA to inquire about the number of MedWatch forms submitted to the FDA on breast implant problems. We were told that they did not know how to access this information as their computer system only records to 500 complaints.)

Lessons for our Future

In November of 2006, the FDA again approved silicone breast implants for general use in the United States after a nearly fifteen-year moratorium.[14] In 1992, the FDA had restricted silicone implants and made them available only to mastectomy patients and other patients under very controlled circumstances because of safety concerns.[15] Although women seeking cosmetic breast augmentation did not have access to silicone implants, saline implants were widely available and

---

[14] United States Center for Disease Control and Prevention. "FDA Approves Silicone Gel-Filled Breast Implants after In-Depth Evaluation." Press release. FDA News. 17 Nov. 2006. 26 Jan. 2009.

[15] Segal, Marian. "A Status Report on Breast Implant Safety." FDA Consumer Magazine. U.S. Food and Drug Administration. November, 1995.

accepted as harmless and safe. Saline implants were considered harmless because if they leak, the saline solution is reabsorbed into the body. Other issues, however, such as the saline liquid's propensity, in some cases, to harbor harmful fungi and bacteria growth were not adequately addressed.

As one of the conditions of approval, the FDA recommended that women opting for silicone implants have periodic breast MRI's in an effort to detect rupture, although the FDA has no means to oversee or enforce this stipulation. As well, it is common knowledge among informed medical professionals that the implants often leak long before they rupture, and that this leakage is not visible on any imaging study, including an MRI.

In my review of the package inserts of all breast implants currently on the market, I saw no mention of chemical or biotoxicity. Several of the implant companies have been notified in court depositions (by myself and others) of the science behind these problems, but so far none of the companies has expressed any interest in coming up with a solution. They seem much more interested in dismissing any scientific evidence as coincidental rather than causative.

I have also personally notified the leadership and the ethics committee of the American Society of Plastic Surgeons and to date they have shown no interest in exploring and making plastic surgeons aware of the problems with breast implants. Instead the ASPS, in a special bulletin released on the day of FDA approval, applauded the return of silicone breast implants to the cosmetic surgery market as a triumph of science.[16] Unfortunately, this "science" is inherently flawed. Many poorly designed "epidemiological studies" were done to eradicate the theory that silicone could be associated with a systemic autoimmune disease.

The review committee of the Institute of Medicine and the FDA ignored large amounts of peer-reviewed literature in other fields such as toxicology.[17] The review committees even ignored research the FDA had funded, which suggested an association between ruptured silicone implants and systemic health issues like fibromyalgia and other connective tissue diseases,[18] even though the results of the study are still posted on the FDA website.[19]

Society as a whole is affected by the failure of its institutions to protect the individual from harm. Whenever

---

[16] "FDA Approves Return of Silicone Breast Implants." Special Joint Bulletin. *The American Society of Plastic Surgeons and The American Society for Aesthetic Plastic Surgery.* 17 November 2006.

[17] Brautbar, Nachman, Andrew Campbell, and Aristo Vojdani, eds. *International Journal of Occupational Medicine and Toxicology.* Special Issue on Silicone Toxicity 4 (1995).

[18] Brown, S. Lori, Gene Pennello, Wendie Anne Berg, Mary Scott Soo, and Michael S. Middleton. "Silicone Gel Breast Implant Rupture, Extracapsular Silicone, and Health Status in a Population of Women." *Journal of Rheumatology* 28 (2001): 996-1003.

[19] "Study of Silicone Gel Breast Implant Rupture, Extracapsular Silicone, and Health Status." *U S Food and Drug Administration.* 29 May 2001. 16 Aug. 2009.
http://www.fda.gov/MedicalDevices/ProductsandMedicalProcedures/Imp lantsandProsthetics/BreastImplants/ucm064382.htm

corporations place profit above safety, and professional organizations ignore scientific research, as well as the human clinical evidence sitting in their exam room, society as a whole is injured. These women, who are seriously ill, do not always regain their health to the degree that allows them to be self-sufficient. If they do not have support systems outside of themselves, most of the silicone gel patients remain on Social Security Disability or Medicaid, and if unable to obtain these resources, are often left homeless with a very poor survival rate.

These women cannot raise their children effectively when they sleep twelve to sixteen hours a day and are in constant, chronic pain. Many of these women have committed suicide, and peer-reviewed studies substantiate that the suicide rate is indeed higher among women with breast implants.[20] Many of these women have sores that are chronically infected all over their bodies from the silicone extruding from the skin.

The majority of these women are severely depressed because of their health condition. My clinical experience is that once the implants begin leaking severely or are ruptured, all patients have adverse health effects. Many of the patients have coping mechanisms which allow them to remain functional and in denial that their silicone gel implants are causing problems, but I frequently hear them

---

[20] Hanes, Allison. "In the Bosom of Death: Suicide Risk Is High among Breast Implant Recipients, Canadian Study Says." *National Post* [Don Mills, Ontario, Canada] 11 Oct. 2006: A22.

express that they regain their energy after explantation, and only then realize how poorly they felt prior to implant removal.

With this in mind, it is my sincere hope that instead of creating another generation of chronically ill women who are unable to maintain careers, raise their children or be productive members of society, that researchers actively pursue alternatives to the current silicone and saline breast implants. It is my sincere hope that these researchers will appreciate the need to avoid the introduction of foreign material and chemicals into the body, for we do not know the long-term effects of these substances on human physiology.

The medical profession has a responsibility to actively support the development of safe implants or augmentation injection procedures in the future, for virtually every plastic surgeon with any experience with breast implants is very familiar with their complications. It is my sincere hope that politics will take a back seat to patient safety in the future investigations by government regulatory agencies.

When we as a society understand how our environment and thoughts influence our collective health, and when we learn to make responsible choices that result in the creation of health rather than disease, then we will be able to avoid choices that cause a segment of our society to fall ill and place unnecessary strain on the society as a whole.

Until we reach a level of consciousness that recognizes that the law of cause and effect (karma) is a universal rather than the local law, we will continue to make shortsighted choices that may be profitable in the immediate future, but very costly in the end. As George Santayana's famous quote goes, "Those who cannot remember the past are condemned to repeat it."[22]

---

[22] Santayana, George. *Life of Reason, Reason in Common Sense.* New York: C. Scribner's Sons, 1905.

Gina's Story

Gina's story begins with asymmetrical breast development in her teenage years. Her first set of implants in 1980 were silicone. She sustained a right rupture seen on a breast MRI and underwent bilateral open capsulectomies with placement of textured saline implants in 1993. She received a diagnosis of lupus in July of 1994. Gina eventually had a right open capsulectomy with removal of her saline implant in 2004, followed by a left open capsulectomy a month later. It is unfortunate that even as a highly educated registered nurse, Gina was not able to avoid complications from both her silicone and later her textured saline implants. She was also not able to avoid misdiagnosis by the medical community.

> "I was born flat-chested . . . but then again, aren't we all? Growing up, I used to pray for pretty, perky boobs . . . NOT! As a teenager, mine looked like pancakes, but worse! One was larger than the other. I was born in 1956, so my high school years were full of halter-tops, low-rise jeans and other revealing clothing (what goes around

comes around again)! I was very self-conscious when wearing bathing suits. Even though my breasts were very small, and I was small (5'6" and 105 pounds), the lopsided appearance really bothered me. In 1980, while trying on bathing suits, I looked at myself in the mirror, and said, 'That's it!' Two weeks later, I had implants.

"I had thought about getting implants for years, dreamed about them, wished for them. What I hadn't done was researched them or heard anything negative about them. I was a registered nurse. You would think that if anything bad was known about surgically implanted devices like implants, I would have heard about it in nursing school, or by working in the hospital or as a healthcare professional, right? WRONG!

"I was a very healthy person. I never got sick. I had been a cheerleader in high school and performed gymnastic stunts. At work, I never called in sick, worked lots of extra shifts to make extra money to buy a home and extras for myself as a single person. That all changed very quickly after receiving the implants.

"Ear infections, pneumonia, skin rashes, frequent sinus infections is how it started. I just felt I was run down from working too much and not getting enough sleep. Eventually I started to notice that my joints were hurting a little. I was the type of person that ignored most aches and pains. I would just take an Advil™ and keep on Truckin'!

"In 1985, I got married. I accepted a position with a company that required extensive travel. I was exhausted on the weekends. It was all I could do to make it home and crawl on the couch and regenerate enough energy for the next week.

"In 1988, I changed jobs so I could stay home more

with my husband and we could start a family. During my first pregnancy, my joints really started to hurt and then my muscles started hurting. Nonetheless, I delivered a healthy boy. Nine months later, I was pregnant again. My second pregnancy was different from the beginning. I felt excruciating pain in all my joints and muscles. I lost that pregnancy. The funny thing was that when the pregnancy was over, I felt like I could run a marathon immediately. Strange!

"Next I began to get frequent infections and occasional rashes. The joint pain and 'cold symptoms' were more frequent. I was sure it was a passing phase that would go away if I just got a chance to rest, which I never did. The years went by and I experienced more joint pain, more muscle pain, and more strange symptoms: blisters in the mouth and nose.

"I had another pregnancy and gave birth in 1994. During that pregnancy, I was in so much pain that I would stay awake at night watching the clock to see when I could take another Tylenol™. When I went to the obstetrician, I complained that I couldn't stand the pain when I lay down on the examining table. He stated that I probably needed to see a rheumatologist after the birth because maybe I had arthritis.

"In the seventh month of the pregnancy I saw an ad for the silicone breast implant Class Action Suit and called the number for more information out of curiosity. That was the first I had heard of anything related to illness and silicone, and I was fixin' to learn a lot! I filled out a questionnaire: yes, yes, yes, yes, yes, yes, yes, yes, yes, yes, yes. I had all the symptoms. It got scary!

"I was ushered right into the lawyer's office. Seeing

this 'DUDE' was enough to scare me, if nothing else! Behind his desk was a painting of him with all kinds of disasters befalling people like car wrecks, airplane crashes, boat crashes, etc. I remembered seeing him on TV saying: 'One call, that's all.' He was the epitome of the classic ambulance chaser. What had I gotten myself into? He was very polite and explained to me that I had quite a few symptoms of silicone toxicity syndrome and needed to be referred to another legal practice for follow up and further medical tests for clarification. I heard what he said, filed it away in my brain as something to follow up on when I was not so busy raising a child, running a corporation and being pregnant...

"I got several calls from them over the next few weeks. Finally, when I was a few weeks postpartum, I went to the physician they referred me to for blood tests and a physical. The results came back positive for Lupus. I took the news as well as could be expected under the circumstances. My exact words were 'Thank God. I'm not nuts! There is a reason for why I'm feeling the way I am! Now, how do we deal with it?'

"The same legal office also referred me to Dr. Susan Kolb. I have to confess that when I first met her I thought she was nutty as a fruitcake. I was used to traditional medicine. I was an RN certified in infusion therapy, nephrology and nursing administration. This woman's treatment includes the laying on of hands? Giving herbs? Come on. The physician I had been using was giving me a different pill for every symptom I had. I was probably on twenty or more different meds when I found Dr. Susan. At one point, I was dangerously near death due to vasculitis of the brain. Under Dr. Susan's care, my condition improved dramatically. I took myself off most of those medications and felt better than I had in a long time.

"Four years ago, however, I had a major setback. I had four surgeries in less than a year. I had extensive surgery for a hysterectomy and repairs from the first pregnancy that weren't done correctly eighteen years before and had gotten worse with age. After the surgery, I had issues with elevated liver enzymes, then a gall bladder removal. Then I had fungal infections in both breasts that necessitated having both my saline implants removed. All this happened within an eleven-month time frame. It was too much for my body to deal with and recovery has been difficult.

"During that time I had to leave my job and was not able to return. I was dragging myself in many days, and I'd have good days and bad. I used to make $100,000 plus a year, and it has definitely hurt our family that I'm not able to work any longer. I've been depressed because of what my illness has put my family through as a result of my inability to bring home an income.

"I had a private disability policy that was supposed to be paying me while I was out ill. I paid my premiums so I thought I'd be paid, right? WRONG! It's been four years and I'm still dealing with that insurance company, trying to obtain the money that was rightfully mine. This has, of course, caused me a great deal of stress. I've been through a lawsuit, repeated mediations and made to suffer repeated insults from lawyers who accuse me of faking it or making up diagnoses. The government disability policy came through after almost four years and was like a miracle!

"The years have now passed: that baby is thirteen

and my older son is eighteen and off to college. I feel blessed that I'm still alive. Some have not been so lucky. As a result of the disease process, and especially becoming friends with Susan AND using her as a healer, I have learned so much about the body's ability to heal itself! God has not given me any more than I can handle, but at times it has been VERY challenging! I have learned that my body is a temple and that I should treat it much better than I did when I put foreign objects into it that wrecked my health.

"Overall, I've learned to count my blessings on a daily basis. I still feel my life is blessed. I have the love of my husband, my children, my family and friends that I can depend on at anytime to do anything for me. I am richer than anyone I know. I am so sorry that those close to me have had to endure the pain of watching me suffer through this horrible silicone implant syndrome. So many do not believe breast implant disease exists, but I've lived through it. I only wish that I'd never gotten the implants when I was twenty-three. What would life have been like, for me, for my family If I had known the dangers of implants?"

-9-
A PRAYER FOR THE WORLD

"Never doubt that a small group of thoughtful committed citizens can change the world: Indeed it's the only thing that ever has."
Margaret Mead

We live in a world in which diseases are progressing at a rate much faster than traditional medical science and research is advancing. Doctors who are clinically investigating these diseases may have the best vantage point to recognize causes and find out which treatments are most successful. For politically incorrect diseases like chronic fatigue syndrome, fibromyalgia, Lyme disease, sick building syndrome and Morgellons disease, doctors who specialize in these areas may risk their medical licenses due to the political climate.

There are tentacles from industry and government that reach into organized medicine to suppress research in these areas. Doctors who dare to publish even in foreign medical journals have had their medical licenses threatened for countering the stance of the vested medical establishment. When money, power and the desire to suppress adverse effects of products and discourage research in controversial areas of medicine exist, it is ultimately the patients who suffer.

If patients do not find a doctor who is willing to step outside the boundaries of traditional medicine, they may not find help that is effective. Public health epidemics of brain tumors, dementia from prion and mad cow disease, disease from weaponized Mycoplasma and other intracellular infectious diseases may be waiting in our not so distant future. The truth regarding the causes of these diseases is being suppressed and treatment is being thwarted. The interference of special interests in the monitoring of these conditions and research into their etiologies will likely be recorded as a failure in medical history.

At an earlier time in our history, hand washing was ridiculed as an ineffective means of decreasing postpartum deaths from infections. Physicians once believed that many diseases were caused by an overabundance of blood in the body, and bloodletting was a common treatment for a variety of ills. This idea, of course, is no longer supported by medical science. I predict that the current treatment of cancer with radiation and chemotherapy will be viewed in a similar manner in the years to come. What we consider advanced technology today will become seen as barbaric as our understanding of health and illness evolves. Meanwhile, the forces of fear and greed block our progress toward creative and innovative solutions to diseases that we encounter.

Ultimately, for medical professionals, it comes down to a simple principle and a choice. You cannot serve two gods. You either serve the god of money and power and protect the government and corporate interests, or you seek the truth despite what it might uncover. For patients, the principles are also clear. To choose security over freedom of choice will severely limit your health options. Many patients with chronic health conditions now seek care outside of the United States for this reason.

For society, allowing the current suppression of research and interference in government regulatory agencies will only increase the burden of the ever growing chronically ill portion of society. This creates a strain on an already economically threatened country. What percentage of our citizens will be on Social Security disability before the entire system collapses?

So in your mind, travel into the future 200 years from now. What do you envision if we do not successfully learn the spiritual lesson that we are all part of the same whole? Do you see children with birth defects, mental illness, young adults unable to produce offspring, a cancer rate that is staggering in its financial and social consequences to society?

Or do you see a world where the precautionary principle and the universal law of cause and effect are understood and respected and a planet that has been cleansed of radiation and chemical contamination, a planet where health and well-being are valued over material profits? One of these two worlds will emerge. The choices we make as a society will steer us into one or the other reality. "As you sow, so shall you reap."

It sounds like a simple concept, but we have forgotten our place in the order of creation. We have also forgotten that our thoughts and our actions today create the world we will inhabit tomorrow. Will we continue on our current path, or will we learn now to choose more wisely?

Will this world be one of suffering, hardship and disease, or will it be one of health, prosperity and freedom? Our prayers should be for wisdom. Our future generations, if they are to exist, depend on our choice.

Index

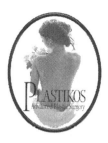

Plastikos Plastic & Reconstructive Surgery
Plastikos Surgery Center
Avatar Industries

Plastikos Surgery Center began as a vision of a healing space where state of the art surgical technology could be combined with compassionate care and holistic healing modalities. Our goal is to ensure that each patient receives the highest quality care while enjoying special attention in a private serene setting. The facility's design features soothing waterfalls, full spectrum lighting, and therapeutic music which helps provide an environment conducive to healing. Plastikos Surgery Center has board certified surgeons and anesthesiologists with state of the art surgical and anesthesia equipment. Plastikos Surgery Center is accredited by the Joint Commission on Accreditation of Healthcare Organizations. This level of accreditation assures that all aspects of your care at Plastikos will be at the highest levels of safety and competence. We are local and nationally accredited. Our center is state licensed (#044-111) and holds the highest level of national accreditation (JCAHO) for an outpatient surgical center. The Joint Commission's Gold Seal of Approval™ and state licensing as well as continued education and growth, demonstrates our commitment to quality care and patient safety.

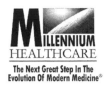

MILLENNIUM
HEALTHCARE
The Next Great Step In The
Evolution Of Modern Medicine®

Millennium Healthcare grants you access to healthcare providers that just don't fight diseases but they strengthen the life force within your body. These providers have an understanding of how spiritual, mental and emotional issues can weaken the life force and allow disease to settle into the physical body. These providers could also help you learn how to strengthen your body's life force system so to not only avoid disease but actually create health and vitality. Millennium Healthcare is different than other holistic centers in that it encompasses the entire range of medicine from surgery to spiritual healing. Many of our practitioners have been practicing holistic medicine for over a decade and draw upon their holistic knowledge and experience to compliment their expertise in western traditional medicine. But unlike many other holistic practitioners, they have a firm understanding of the benefits of traditional medicine and are licensed to use it when appropriate.

MedSpa

Our philosophy at Plastikos MedSpa is to provide our clients with state of the art non-surgical enhancement treatments in a relaxing spa environment. Our goal is beauty through health and relaxation to restore what life extracts from us on a daily basis. Individual customized treatments are vital in reaching this goal. Our wide variety of treatments and our holistic approach enables us to provide you with a multitude of choices to best suit your needs.

Our Physicians and Medical Estheticians specialize in skincare, detoxification, anti-aging, skin rejuvenation, microcurrent technology to include inch loss (Ion Magnum) and non-surgical face lift (Perfector), Lipomassage by Endermologie and spa essentials to promote a healthier lifestyle throughout the mind, body, and soul.